Overcoming Social Anxiety and Building Self-confidence:

A Self-help Guide for Teenagers

Eleanor Leigh, Emma Warnock-Parkes,
Elyse Brassard and David M. Clark

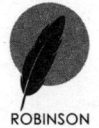

ROBINSON

ROBINSON

First published in Great Britain in 2024 by Robinson

13 5 7 9 10 8 6 4 2

Copyright © Eleanor Leigh, Emma Warnock-Parkes,
Elyse Brassard and David M. Clark, 2024
Photos on pp. 70, 105, and 243 and images on pp 81, 290 and 291 © iStock
All other illustrations by Liane Payne

The moral rights of the authors have been asserted.

Important Note
This book is not intended as a substitute for medical advice or treatment.
Any person with a condition requiring medical attention should consult
a qualified medical practitioner or suitable therapist.

A CIP catalogue record for this book
is available from the British Library.

ISBN: 978-1-47214-741-7

Typeset in Palatino by Initial Typesetting Services, Edinburgh
Printed and bound in Great Britain by Clays Ltd, Elcograf S.p.A.

Papers used by Robinson are from well-managed forests and other
responsible sources.

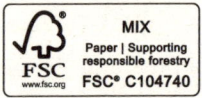

Robinson
An imprint of
Little, Brown Book Group
Carmelite House
50 Victoria Embankment
London EC4Y 0DZ

An Hachette UK Company
www.hachette.co.uk

www.littlebrown.co.uk

INTRODUCING US

Eleanor Leigh

Dr Eleanor Leigh is an Associate Professor at the Department of Experimental Psychology, University of Oxford. Her work focuses on the understanding and treatment of anxiety problems in young people.

Emma Warnock-Parkes

Dr Emma Warnock-Parkes is a Clinical Psychologist at the Oxford Centre for Anxiety Disorders and Trauma, University of Oxford. As part of an internationally recognised research group, Emma specialises in the development and evaluation of treatments for social anxiety and other anxiety disorders.

Elyse Brassard

Elyse is a student at the University of Manchester studying psychology and is originally from London. Elyse writes as an expert by lived experience.

David M. Clark

Professor David M. Clark is an Emeritus Professor of Experimental Psychology at the University of Oxford. He is well known for his ground-breaking research on the understanding and treatment of anxiety related disorders, including social anxiety, panic disorder, health anxiety and post-traumatic stress. Recognition of his work includes Lifetime Achievement Awards from the British Psychological Society and the American Psychological Association.

Overcoming for Teenagers is a series to support young people through common mental health issues during adolescence, using scientific techniques that have been proven to work.

Series editors: Associate Professor Polly Waite and Emeritus Professor Peter Cooper.

Titles in the series include:

Overcoming Worries about Body Image and Eating

Contents

Welcome from the Authors

Almost all of us feel anxious about embarrassing ourselves in front of other people from time to time, and especially when we are teenagers. While these worries are mild for most people, for some they are more troublesome and persistent.

We wrote this evidence-based book for young people who are struggling with social anxiety and for their families. Although it may feel difficult now, social anxiety can improve with the right help. You might be considering accessing help, waiting for treatment or perhaps you would just like to feel a bit more confident in your relationships and at school or college.

This book will help you understand what keeps social anxiety going and provide key steps to building self-confidence. There are also additional sections on common fears, including the fear of being stared at, the fear of blushing, shaking or sweating, feeling boring, stupid, unlikeable or weird. You will also find chapters on being kinder to yourself and managing social media, teasing or bullying, and friendships.

We hope you find this book helps build your social confidence. But you might find that you would like more active support. If so, then the first step is to speak to a teacher or your family doctor. They can help you to access treatment. If you are sixteen years old or over you may be able to access help directly (called 'self-referral'). The treatment you are offered should be a psychological (or 'talking') therapy. Commonly this might be cognitive behavioural therapy ('CBT' for short), which usually involves meeting a therapist weekly for two to three months, learning about anxiety and how to overcome it. CBT has been shown to work well for the treatment of social anxiety.

Good luck!

Chapter 1

Getting Started

What is social anxiety?

> Going to a party
>
> Answering a question in class
>
> Being the centre of attention

How does the thought of being in these situations make you feel?

Anxious? Stressed? Do you dread the thought of your name being called in class, of all eyes turning on you?

If you answered 'yes' to any of the above, then this book is for you. We will get started in this chapter by learning about:

- What social anxiety is

- Why some people experience social anxiety

- How this book can help

Why do these situations cause anxiety? Behind the anxiety is a fear of doing something that will be embarrassing and of being judged by other people:

I've got nothing to say; people will think I'm boring.

I'll blush and everyone will laugh at me.

I will look nervous, and everyone will know it.

Such worries are normal. Friendships are important to most of us and so it makes sense that we can get preoccupied by our relationships.

The worries are often strongest when we are teenagers. When we are little, we might worry about monsters, about dogs, about being separated from our parents, but as we move into secondary school and college and become more independent from our family and reliant on our friends, we worry about building relationships, connections with people around us and being accepted by others.

For most people, the worries bubble up as we move into adolescence, and then fade away with time, without getting in the way of day-to-day life. But for some people, the worries take hold and affect how we feel and what we do. The anxiety can be so strong that it gets in the way of day-to-day life and causes distress. We call this social anxiety.

Understandably, social anxiety can lead people to try to avoid situations they fear. This might be turning down an invitation to a party, not putting your hand up in class or staying silent in a group text conversation.

But because it is difficult to avoid contact with others altogether, often people will get through the situations they fear 'with gritted teeth'. They will endure the situation, hoping to 'fly under the radar' and avoid being noticed and judged.

Do you recognise the description above? Does it sound like you? If you answered yes to that, you are not alone. Social anxiety is the most common kind of anxiety. Take a moment to picture an average classroom with thirty students. Then consider that five of those students will be experiencing some difficulty with social anxiety.

Elyse's reflections

Hiya! I'm Elyse and I'm someone who at one point had pretty severe social anxiety. It didn't seem so to others because I was good at masking my anxiety, but it seriously sucked and I felt terrible almost all the time. For me, social anxiety was at its worst when I was between fourteen and sixteen years old. I saw people around me forming new friendships and hanging out and I suddenly felt incompetent compared to them. My anxieties impacted how I interacted with others, made me turn down good opportunities like taking up the offer of careers advice from school, and took a toll on my grades. I very quickly shut myself away mentally to stop myself from feeling this way. The worst part is that no one seemed to realise how much I was struggling – I had trained myself to appear 'normal', and although it helped me momentarily in brief social situations, it did nothing but make me feel worse about myself because I felt like everything I was doing was fake. All the interactions I had with my friends and family felt surface level, and it just sucked a whole bunch.

These feelings obviously were not good for my mood – I often felt depressed and isolated – it affected my appetite and my sleep schedule. I was more reserved with my family and it felt like I spent most of my days spaced out – barely even registering the things and people around me.

After getting sick and tired of feeling terrible constantly, I started to make changes to the way I approached different aspects of my life. I made the changes through a kind of therapy called cognitive behavioural therapy, and the techniques you will learn about in this book are all taken from this therapy. In therapy I learnt to be kind to myself but also firm: I had to be able to acknowledge that this was a part of me and that my feelings were valid, but that I had to be proactive if I wanted to get out of this rut. Now, I can listen to myself and trust myself, I don't worry about what other people think of me. I have left home and I am studying at university. In this book I'll be giving my perspective, which I hope you find helpful.

As well as hearing from Elyse, we will hear the stories of two young people who have struggled with their social confidence. We will follow their journeys through the book. Let's meet them:

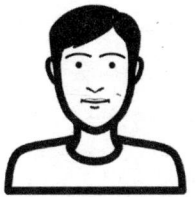

JOSH

Josh is a fifteen-year-old boy. He likes playing football and his favourite school subject is geography. From the outside, it seems like things are going OK for Josh.

In reality, he is finding life really difficult. He is anxious about how he comes across to other people. He finds it hard to think about anything else and he feels like he is walking about with this anxiety all the time.

Josh is scared of speaking to people he doesn't know well, of going to parties and of chatting in groups.

He dreads break times at school most because this is when everyone hangs around in groups and chats. He becomes anxious whenever break or lunch approaches.

When the bell rings, he tags along at the back of his group of classmates and thinks:

> *What am I going to say? . . . I can't think of anything to say. Why am I so boring? The others will be wondering why I'm here and not want to talk to me. Why am I like this?*

Josh notices his heart beating fast, his head is swirling.

He stays on the edge of the group and avoids eye contact in the hope that no one will speak to him.

When he does have to speak to someone, he monitors how he is coming across and rehearses what he is going to say before he says it. He holds back from saying things that he worries other people might find boring. When he has finished speaking, he glues his eyes to the ground and hopes no one else will ask him a question.

When the bell rings and break is over, Josh feels embarrassed and angry with himself for finding such a simple thing so difficult.

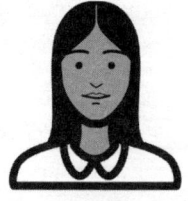

NITA

Nita is a sixteen-year-old girl in her first year at college. She likes playing computer games and reading graphic novels, and she is studying art, philosophy and sociology.

Nita hates being the centre of attention. She can't bear answering or asking questions in class. She avoids speaking up in a group, preferring to speak one-to-one.

She gets most stressed out when she has to give a presentation in class.

Recently, Nita had to give a presentation to her sociology class. She thought:

> *I'm not as confident as the others . . . Will they notice? . . . Will I blush? . . . Will I shake? . . . I look nervous and weird.*

As she thought this, she began to feel hot, and felt that she must be looking flustered and blushing. Her hands felt shaky. She could picture how she must look to the class – really red and shaky, just a weird mess – which made her feel even more embarrassed.

Nita gripped her paper tightly; she avoided looking at the other students and rushed to get her presentation finished. She let her hair fall down over her face to try to cover her blush. When she sat down again, she felt mortified.

You have probably looked at other people who seem more confident and wished you could be like them. Maybe you have hoped that the worries would go away with time but they haven't. The good news is that social anxiety can be overcome. Our team has spent many years developing powerful evidence-based tools to help people free themselves from social anxiety. In this book we will walk you through the key steps to doing this. By starting this book, you have begun your journey to overcome social anxiety and build your social confidence.

Let's begin by looking at how you would like things to be different by the end of this book.

What do I want to change?

As you answer this question, remember that we all feel a bit anxious and worry about what others think of us sometimes. For example, it is totally natural to feel a little nervous about giving a presentation. In other words, it isn't realistic to imagine we could feel *no* anxiety! A life without anxiety isn't possible and wouldn't be good either – anxiety can act as an alarm system to alert us to danger and keep us safe. When you are thinking about what you would like to change, it can be more helpful to think about what anxiety stops you doing:

- What do you find difficult because of the feelings of anxiety?

- What would you **like** to do that anxiety gets in the way of?

- What is **important** to you to do that is difficult because of anxiety?

Try to be as detailed as possible – the more specific the goals, the better we can reach them!

As you make your goals, you might ask yourself these questions:

- What bothers you most about your anxiety?

- How would you like things to be different?

- What would you like to be able to do, that you don't do now (or find difficult) because of your anxiety?

- What would you like to achieve in the short and long term?

Here are Josh's goals:

GOAL 1: To chat to classmates at break time in school and with the other players at football, without all the stress and without holding back.

GOAL 2: To go to parties. I turn down invitations or, if I do go, I turn up with people and leave as soon as I can. My goal would be to enjoy a full party.

GOAL 3: To speak confidently to strangers and people I don't know well. In the short term, I want to feel comfortable speaking to shop assistants, school staff and people like that. In the long term I want to feel comfortable meeting people when I leave school in the summer and take up training or a job.

Here are Nita's goals:

GOAL 1: To answer and ask questions in class.

GOAL 2: To give presentations in class.

GOAL 3: To speak up in groups and to celebrate my birthday with a group of friends this year (I've always avoided this because I find the thought of being the centre of attention too uncomfortable).

GOAL 4: To allow people to take photos of me and upload selfies without filtering and editing.

What are your goals? Write these down here or in a notebook or the notes section of your phone. You can write as many goals as you like. You might want to write your top three goals below.

My goals are:

GOAL 1: _____

_____

_____

GOAL 2: _____

_____

_____

GOAL 3: _____

_____

_____

We will revisit your goals at the end of the book to see how much progress you have made towards them.

Why me?

You might have found yourself wondering, *Why me? Why do I find social situations so stressful?* Nobody knows the answer to this for sure, but it is likely to be a combination of genetics and life experiences. There are several reasons why people develop social anxiety:

You might recognise some of these for you.

Biology and temperament: We are born with genes that make us more or less likely to experience social anxiety. Part of the reason why some people tend to be more socially anxious is to do with their genes.

Were you always quite shy? Perhaps you have always been the kind of person who likes to take their time, to familiarise themselves with a new situation before exploring. But you might notice that some of your friends or classmates seem to approach life differently. There are those who are always up for things, keen to explore, to try new things and have a go. We know that people vary in how shy/inhibited, outgoing/ exploratory they are. This seems to be linked to our temperament (or personality) and it is evident from early on in life. For example, if you were to go into any nursery or reception class at primary school, you would see that some children rush in and start playing with the toys and interacting straight away, while others hang back, holding close to their parent's legs, scoping out what is going on before they ease themselves into the activity. Research has shown us that there is a link between being inhibited as a child and going on to feel socially anxious; for some people who are more inhibited they may be more likely to experience social anxiety, particularly if they are faced with difficult life experiences.

Difficult experiences: The particular experiences we have can also explain why some people experience social anxiety. Research suggests that nega- 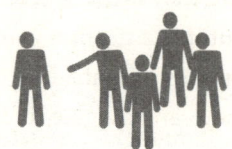 tive experiences, perhaps particularly negative social experiences like being bullied, may make some people more likely to develop social anxiety.

Looking back, were there any difficult experiences you went through that relate to your social confidence? Some people with social anxiety recall being bullied, gossiped about, left out or treated differently to others. Others remember finding the transition to secondary school challenging and this coinciding with an uptick in their social anxiety. Research has found a link between difficult life experiences, particularly those that relate to other people, and later social anxiety.

Home life: Things to do with our home environment, like how we are parented, may partly 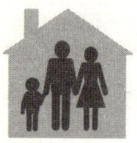 explain why some people develop social anxiety.

Parents bring their own anxieties and worries to the job of parenting. Some parents feel so worried about their children that they can tend to 'overprotect', like not giving their child the freedoms that would be expected given their age. For example, they may not allow them to go on trips with their friends. Some parents might feel anxious for their child in social situations, so they might interfere or speak for their child. These kinds of reactions are understandable because parents themselves might struggle with worry and shyness and they are trying to do their best to care for their children. But it can mean a young person doesn't get as many opportunities to learn how the world works and to discover that they can navigate it.

It can be helpful to make sense of where a lack of social confidence came from, especially if you are bothered by the 'Why me?' question.

But there is an even more important question to answer than **Why me?** And that is **What keeps my anxiety going?** If we know what keeps anxiety going, then we can break the chain and build confidence.

So that is what we will focus on in this book: understanding what is driving your anxiety and learning to do things differently in social situations.

Elyse's reflections

I'd always been quite quiet but primary school had been OK. I had some friends and did all right in school. But my social anxiety started from about age eleven onwards, around the time I went to secondary school. Everything felt different with the change. Other people seemed to manage it well and I saw my friends from primary school making new friendships and groups. I didn't know how to fit in and I found it hard to connect to others. It felt really isolating and I got more and more anxious.

How can this book help me?

As you will read more about in the next chapter, what we think and what we do when we feel anxious in social situations keeps anxiety going. This means that we can get locked in a vicious cycle in which our thoughts affect our feelings, what we do and how we see ourselves.

This book will help you to spot your unhelpful thoughts and to understand how they affect how you feel and what you do. You will then learn how to see yourself in a positive light and to feel confident in who you are.

How can I get the most out of this book?

How do we learn any new skill, whether that is how to cook, play a musical instrument or a new sport?

First we learn the basics, through reading or in person, and then we apply what we have learnt in practice. To fine-tune those skills, we need to continue practising over time.

In just the same way, the best way to build your social confidence with this book is by investing some time to achieving the goals you set yourself.

Top Tips

★ Set aside some time to read this book on a regular basis. Perhaps you could schedule some dedicated time to do this on the calendar of your phone.

★ Fill in the boxes with your own experiences. Either you can complete the boxes in the book or you could do it in the notes section on your phone or in a notebook.

★ Give the activities a go. Some of the tasks will feel difficult at first, and this is to be expected; if they were easy then you wouldn't need this book. The more you can try the ideas out in action, the more quickly your confidence will grow.

★   Some people find it helpful to ask a family member or close friend to support them as they work through the book. Do you think that might help you? Who could be a good support?

★   Give yourself credit as you work through the book. It can be easy to overlook small achievements or beat yourself up if you aren't making progress as quickly as you would like. But remember it will take a while to learn new 'confident' habits. Give yourself the support you would give a friend on this journey: praise efforts just as much as successes and be kind in the face of setbacks.

We encourage you to work your way through the book from start to finish in the order it is presented. This is because some of the later chapters will build on ideas that are introduced earlier on.

Elyse's reflections

It's not something that you can just read once and have all the skills. You have to put it into practice and put the effort in and actively make those changes. It is worth the effort!

Key points and giving yourself credit

 You've finished the first chapter. This is the first step towards tackling your anxiety and reaching your goals. Throughout the book we encourage you to pause after each chapter and give yourself some credit for your achievements, however small. It can also help to make a note of your key learning points. You can do this in this book, in your own notebook or on a phone/device – whatever works best for you.

For example, Nita wrote:

What I can give myself credit for	Key learning points
Reading this chapter for starters has been a big step for me.	Social anxiety is common. Five kids in a class is more than I thought. It is good to know I am not the only one.
Writing some goals in my notebook.	There are several causes of social anxiety. For me, it is probably a mix of my genetics along with some teasing I had when I was younger.
	What is more important is learning what fuels my anxiety now, as I can change those things. It felt good to write some goals and I feel hopeful that things can change if I work on my anxiety.

Do you agree with Nita's thoughts on giving herself credit and her learning points? If there is anything else you would like to add you can put it in the table below.

What I can give myself credit for	Key learning points

In the next chapter, we will find out what keeps your social anxiety going so that we can learn how to overcome it.

Chapter 2

Understanding My Social Anxiety

Well done for starting this chapter and taking another step forward in building your social confidence. In the next few pages we will:

- Learn what drives social anxiety

- Map out our anxiety to start us on the path to overcoming it

---

Elyse's reflections

I used to feel as though there was something wrong with me, and everyone could see it. It felt like I stood out, like everybody was looking at me constantly – and they were about to make fun of me. It was only when I started to map out my anxiety that I realised it was my thoughts and behaviours that were keeping it going. I recommend you give mapping your anxiety a go. You may feel stuck right now, but having a clear idea of what was driving my anxiety allowed me to figure out the next steps to take.

Anxiety overdrive

Some of my friends don't seem to care about talking in front of others – why does it make me *feel so nervous? –* Nita

It's normal to feel anxious from time to time – everyone does. So why is your anxiety in overdrive?

Cognitive behavioural therapy, which is what this book is based on, is a talking therapy that helps people overcome social anxiety. It is based on the tried-and-tested theory that the way we think about social situations affects how we feel, what we pay attention to and what we do. Some of the thoughts you have in social situations may make you feel anxious and impact what you focus on and the way you behave.

Let's take Nita as an example. When Nita finds herself in a group, she has **negative thoughts** like, *I'm shaking and red* or, *I look weird*. The thoughts make her feel **anxious and self-conscious**. She starts to focus on herself and on how she is coming across. She is watching herself, monitoring herself and imagining how she might appear to others. When the **spotlight of her attention turns inwards**, she is really aware of how shaky and hot she feels. The more she focuses on herself, the more self-conscious and anxious she feels. She starts to picture herself looking red and shaky and thinks, *Others will notice and think I look anxious*. At this point she looks down to avoid eye contact with her friends and she keeps quiet. These strategies (**behaviour traps**) make her feel even more self-conscious because they keep her locked in her head, checking that the strategies are working. She then makes an excuse to leave, worrying, *I looked so weird. They won't want to know me.* Nita finds herself stuck in a vicious cycle: her negative thoughts driving her anxiety, how she saw herself and then what she did in the situation:

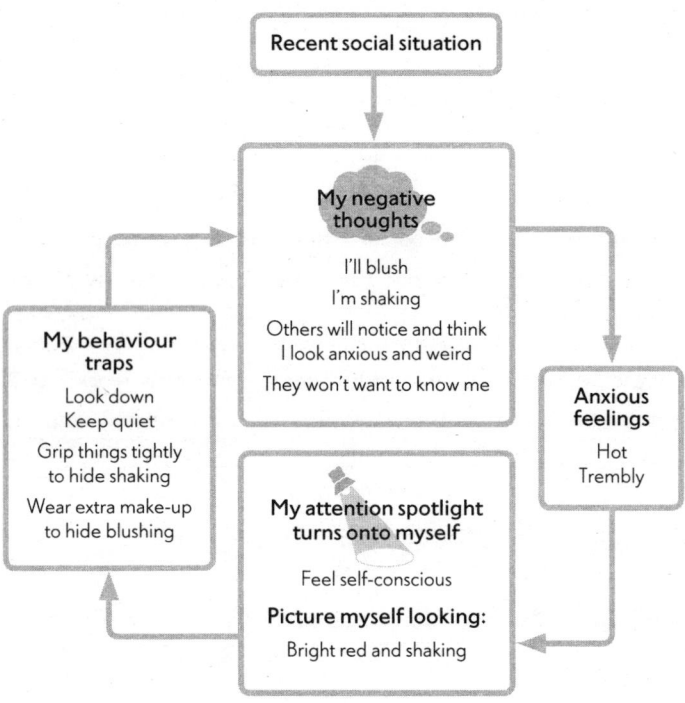

Before we see how this vicious cycle might work for you, let's find out more about these three driving forces in social anxiety: our (1) negative thoughts, (2) self-focused attention and (3) behaviour traps.

1. The danger comes from our thoughts

If you were asked to give a talk in class and had the thought, *I can do that, no problem,* how would you feel? You might feel OK to step up. But when we suffer with social anxiety our thoughts tend to jump to the negative instead.

'I'll freeze!'   'I'll look anxious'

It will be really awkward'   'People will stare and think I'm an idiot.'

'I'll say something boring or stupid'   'I'll embarrass myself'

Do any of these sound familiar? When our thoughts jump to the negative our brain detects danger, so our body reacts as it does when it sees danger – with anxiety.

When Josh talks to others he thinks, *I have nothing to say. Everybody thinks I'm boring.* So it makes sense that he feels nervous at school, meeting friends or going to parties. Everybody worries about what others think sometimes. But some of us have more negative thoughts about how we come across than others. Which of the following are most common for you?

Negative thoughts about doing or saying something that you think others will judge:

❏ I'll have nothing to say

❏ I'll say something boring

❑ I'll say something stupid

❑ My mind will go blank

❑ I won't make any sense

❑ I'll look anxious

❑ I'll blush

❑ I'll shake

❑ I'll sweat

Negative thoughts about yourself and how you come across overall:

❑ I'm unlikeable

❑ I'm boring

❑ I'm stupid

❑ I'm not good enough

❑ I'm weird/different/odd

Negative thoughts about how others might react:

❑ People won't want to be friends with me

❑ People are not interested in me

❑ People will stare at me

❑ People will laugh at me or make fun of me

❑ People will be angry with me

Look back at any thoughts you ticked above. If these things were going through anybody's head in a social situation, would it make sense that they were feeling anxious or self-conscious?

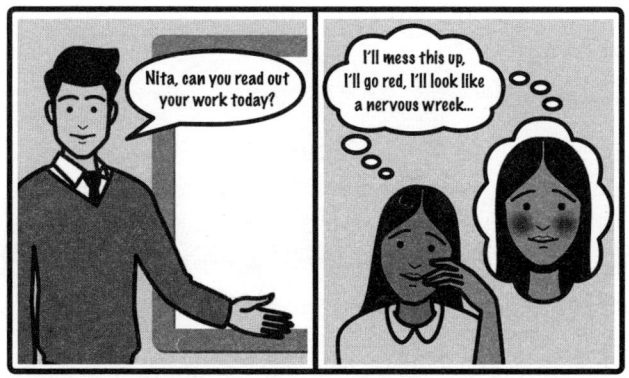

Negative thoughts are a key driving force in our social anxiety. Thankfully, although they feel true at the time, our **thoughts *are not* facts**. This is a key message you will discover as you work through this book.

2. Self-focused attention and the spotlight effect

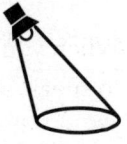

I feel so self-conscious when I speak, like all eyes are on me and it's painful – Josh

---

Elyse's reflections

A big problem for me was that I was so self-conscious and super aware of myself. It felt like everybody was staring at me. I see now that this came from being so focused on the way I was appearing. I constantly asked myself, *How am I sounding? How am I looking? Am I making too much eye contact? Is it normal the way I am holding my hands or the way I'm sitting?* I'd get so focused on the way I appear, and I'd lose sight of the actual conversation itself. I was staring at myself and mistakenly thinking other people were staring at me in the same way, but they weren't.

When feeling anxious in social situations it can feel like we are centre stage and under the spotlight – like all eyes are on us. If you often feel self-conscious, you are not alone. It may *feel* like we are standing out, but are we really? Research carried out at our clinic at the University of Oxford shows that socially anxious people overestimate how many people are staring at them. But why is this? The answer lies in what we are most focused on in social situations.

When you walk into a party or step up in front of your class to speak, are you:

A) Totally lost in what everybody else is doing and saying?

or

B) More focused on yourself, how you are feeling and coming across to others?

When feeling socially anxious, we tend to turn the spotlight of our attention onto **ourselves**. When we start to watch ourselves too closely it feels like everybody else is doing the same. **It feels like you are in the spotlight, but the only person watching you that closely is you.**

Do any of the following things apply to you?

In social situations that I find difficult:

❑ I feel self-conscious

❑ I'm focused on myself and how I'm coming across

❑ I'm often stuck in my own head

❑ I'm more focused on myself than the situation

Putting our feelings under the spotlight

The problem with focusing on ourselves is that this can make us feel more nervous and self-conscious. The other problem is that when we focus on ourselves and our feelings this tends to fuel a negative sense or image of how we think we look to others.

Remember Nita – when she speaks up in class **she focuses on** how hot and shaky she feels **and then pictures herself** looking like a red and shaky mess.

When Josh meets up with a group of friends **he focuses on** how boring he feels **and then he gets an impression** of himself as looking dull.

Nita and Josh have a negative self-image or impression that comes from focusing so much on how they feel. This then makes them more convinced that they are coming across badly. This makes them both even more anxious – the vicious cycle continues.

The good news is that we may not look as bad as we feel. Your feelings are private and only you know how you are feeling on the inside. Think about the last person you spoke to – how quickly was their heart beating? How shaky did their hands feel? This is information you do not know because it is private to the other person and not visible on the outside.

When you listen to music through your headphones, you hear the music, and you might feel the bass vibrating, but other people around cannot hear it. The same goes for your thoughts and feelings in social situations. You might notice your heart racing and feel hot, but others cannot see or hear what is going on inside your body. **Your thoughts and feelings are private.**

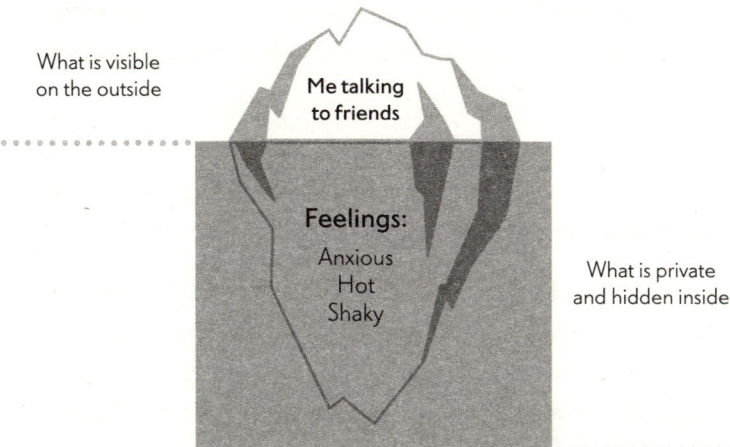

What is visible on the outside

Me talking to friends

Feelings:
Anxious
Hot
Shaky

What is private and hidden inside

This book is all about teaching you how to **stop putting yourself under the spotlight and start getting out of your head.** We want you to start seeing yourself in just the same way other people do. This will help you enjoy your social life more and feel calmer – win, win!

3. Our behaviours are a trap

In situations we find scary, we do things to keep ourselves safe. If we think we will be humiliated, embarrassed or end up without friends, it makes sense that we might do things to try to hide the parts of ourselves that we don't want others to see. The problem is that some of the things we do can backfire and keep our anxiety going. Let's find out more about the types of behaviour traps we can get stuck in.

Avoidance and hiding: Sometimes we might avoid things altogether, like saying no to an invitation from friends. Even if we do go, we might try to hide ourselves when we are there by keeping quiet or not saying much about ourselves.

Putting on a performance: Perhaps it feels like conversations are a performance, rather than a chance to just hang out with others. We might try to come across better to others, like only saying things we think sound cool, clever or interesting, rather than just going with the flow.

Behaviour traps can stop us being our true selves and, as a result, we never end up discovering we are OK as we are. Here are some of the other ways these behaviours can trap us:

- **They stop us finding out we come across better than we think:** Take Nita, who worries about blushing. She rarely speaks up in groups or class. She wears extra make-up to hide blushing and looks down if she feels hot in the face. Keeping quiet and looking down means she never finds out what her friends do when she feels she is blushing. If she were to look up, she might see her friends carrying on as normal and find out her blush is barely noticeable.

  Josh thinks he's boring, so he plans interesting things to talk to his friends about. Even if a meet-up goes well, he feels like he was only liked because he thought about fun things to say in advance. He never feels accepted for himself.

- **They can impact on our conversations and relation-ships with others:** Owing to Nita's worries about appearing anxious, she tries to avoid being the centre of attention. She usually turns down invitations to parties or meet-ups because of her fear. But this just gives her friends the impression that she is not interested in meeting up and over time they stop inviting her to things.

During conversations, Josh is busy thinking about what he is going to say and making sure it sounds interesting. This makes it hard for him to follow any chat because he's too busy thinking about what he is going to say and, as a result, he is not really listening to his friends. This sometimes means that Josh sits very quietly and does not say much at all. His friends often think this means he is not interested in them. The message they pick up is the opposite to the one he wants to give. He also judges himself as boring because he didn't speak very much. But remember, Josh had in some senses chosen not to speak very much (it is one of his behaviour traps).

• **They can make some of the things we are worried about happen more:** Nita also worries about shaking. When she feels shaky, she grips her cup super-tight to try to stop her arm from shaking. This backfires because when we hold something tightly it can make our muscles feel more trembly (give it a go if you're curious!).

Josh spends so long in his head trying to think of things to say he then finds it hard to say anything at all when in a group – which is one of his worst fears.

Overall, our behaviour traps make us feel more anxious and self-conscious and lead to more negative thoughts about how we are coming across. In the book we will learn how to drop our behaviour traps to help us feel more confident.

Elyse's reflections

My behaviour traps (like planning and overthinking everything I said to people) meant I wasn't able to focus on what the others were saying in conversations. I would forget what they said or I wouldn't be able to respond properly. I wasn't really engaged in the conversation. Without my behaviour traps now I'm less self-conscious about the way that I'm appearing to others. I'm able to just focus more on the conversation, on what they're saying. I can listen to what they're saying and share my actual opinion of things. Not doing that before made me feel like I wasn't being a real person, and that made me feel even more isolated.

Which of the following strategies are most common for you?

Things I do to avoid being noticed:

❑   Plan excuses or a 'get out'

❑   Try to look busy

❑   Talk less

❏ Stay on the edge of things

❏ Wear clothes that won't draw attention from others

❏ Get other people to speak or do things for me

Things I do to try to come across better:

❏ Try to come across normal

❏ Try to come across well

❏ Think of interesting or clever things to say

When I'm worried about things I say I:

❏ Rehearse sentences in my mind

❏ Check what I am going to say

❏ Avoid pauses

❏ Prepare things to say in advance

When I'm worried about appearing anxious I:

❏ Wear make-up or cover my face to hide blushing

❏ Wear dark clothes or layers to hide sweat

❏ Grip things tightly or try to control shaking

Take a moment to think about some of the behaviour traps you ticked above. Like you saw with Nita and Josh, could any of these be backfiring in any way? If so, do not be hard on yourself, you have done really well to spot it. In later chapters, we cover how to deal with behaviour traps that do not help us, so we can start to be ourselves more with others. This is the route to feeling accepted for yourself and feeling more confident.

Mapping my own vicious cycle

Now it is time to map out your own social anxiety cycle. Having a road map of what is keeping your social anxiety going is a step forward in overcoming it. We will now walk through the three key steps of mapping your social anxiety.

1. My negative thoughts and feelings

Think about a recent social situation that you found difficult. For example, registration time at school, a meet-up with friends, participating in class, a party you went to or a talk in class. Try to think of a situation that you stayed in for some time, rather than one you left immediately. Ask yourself:

- What was going through my mind at the time?

- Was I worried I might do or say something that might embarrass me?

- Did I have any negative thoughts about myself and how I was coming across?

- What did I worry others were thinking?

Now make a note of the thoughts you had in this situation in box 1 on the chart on page 37. You can also do this on a bit of paper or on notes on your phone. To help spot key thoughts, look back at the checklist earlier in the chapter and note down those that applied to you on your map.

With all those thoughts in your mind, ask yourself, *What was the impact of the thoughts on my feelings?* Were you feeling calm or increasingly anxious? If you were feeling anxious, add signs of anxiety you noticed in your body in the box labelled 'anxious feelings' (e.g. feeling hot, heart racing, feeling shaky). Hopefully you can see that your negative thoughts may have been driving your anxious feelings. Next let's look at what happened to your attention spotlight.

2. My spotlight of attention and how I imagine myself

When you were worried about how you were coming across and feeling anxious, what was happening to your focus of attention? Were you lost in what others were doing or saying? Or were you more focused on yourself and how you were feeling? As the spotlight of your attention turned on to yourself, did you notice feeling self-conscious? Did you feel like you stood out?

As you felt self-conscious – how did you picture the way you came across to others? Did you have a negative image of yourself? Did you have an impression of how you thought you came across? If you had to describe this image or impression to somebody, how would you say you looked in this situation? Make a note of how you saw yourself coming across in box 3 on the chart opposite.

Hopefully you can see that focusing on yourself fuels your negative self-image – it can make it feel more real. Now let's look at what you understandably did in this situation.

3. *My behaviour traps*

When you were thinking in this negative way, feeling anxious and self-conscious, was there anything you were going to try to keep safe or prevent your fears being noticed? Ask yourself:

- Was I trying to hide myself in any way? If so, how?

- Did I do anything to try to hide how I was feeling?

- Did I do anything to make a good impression, to come across well?

Make a note of anything you were doing in box 3 on the chart opposite. It might help to look back at the checklist of behaviour traps earlier in this chapter and add any that apply. Take a moment to consider what impact these traps might have had. Is it possible that doing some of these things might have kept some of your negative thinking about yourself going or made you feel more self-conscious?

My social anxiety map

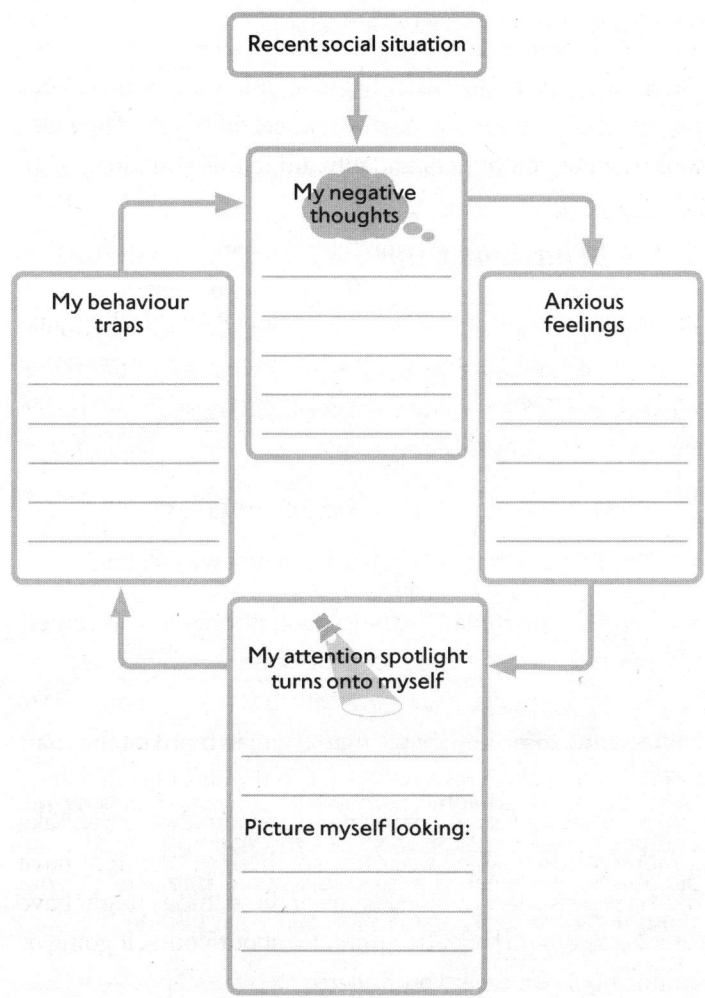

Your own worst enemy?

What you will see above is what happens during social situations. Like many other people, you may also find that afterwards you end up dissecting everything you just said and did. That your thoughts become your own worst enemy. Going over and over things can make us feel low, ashamed, more anxious, embarrassed or cross. It can fuel our negative thoughts about ourselves too. The more we overthink things we think we messed up, the more we are convinced other people are doing the same. But the chances are they have moved on with their day. This book will cover how to stop this inner bully or inner critic and start being a better friend to yourself.

Taking it forward

This is not an easy task, so well done for giving it a go. Hopefully mapping your own cycle has helped you start to understand some key things that drive your anxiety.

Over the week to come it might help to try mapping out another social situation, to see if this cycle applies. In social situations this week, try to notice what happens to your thoughts, your focus of attention and what you do.

In this book we walk you through step by step how to deal with your negative thoughts, self-focused attention and behaviour traps. We will use tried-and-tested tools to help reduce your social anxiety and build your confidence.

Take action

Try this exercise: What is helping me and what is holding me back?

To find out more about what is keeping your social anxiety going, we suggest you try an exercise we have done many hundreds of times in our clinic. People tell us this really helps them discover for themselves how their social anxiety works. That it helps them to see the path forward to feeling more confident. You could try this yourself the next time you speak to somebody else. It only takes a few minutes. Remember that testing out ideas and trying them out for yourself is the best way to learn.

The 3 key steps are:

1.   When talking to somebody, speak for one to two minutes while being in your own head thinking about how you are coming across. Ask yourself, *How interesting do I sound? How clever?* Think carefully about every word you say.

2.   Then, switch this around. For the next one to two minutes try to get totally lost in the chat and focus more on the other person than on yourself. Focus on how they look, what they say. Rather than thinking about what you say, just say whatever comes to mind. Don't overthink it.

3.   After the conversation, compare the two ways of speaking. In which did you feel more anxious? In which did you feel more self-conscious? Which did you enjoy more?

Most people find that they feel more anxious and more self-conscious when they are more in their head and focusing on themselves. They also feel better and enjoy the chat more when they are out of their head and more focused on the other person.

> *Josh tried this task to find out more about what was keeping his social anxiety going. The next time he met up with his friend he spent the first minute or two focusing on himself. He carefully planned everything he was going to say, asking himself, How boring do I sound? He found himself feeling nervous and on edge. After a couple of minutes, he switched to doing things differently. Instead of focusing on himself, he tried to get lost in what his friend was saying and tried saying whatever came into his mind. Josh found this hard at first, but after a couple of minutes he felt more comfortable and less anxious. He didn't feel quite as boring. This was a key discovery for Josh – his anxiety was driven by being too much in his head.*

Why don't you give this a go now? Once you have tried it out for yourself, you might want to make a few notes on what you learnt.

When I focused on myself . . .

When I focused on the conversation . . .

What I learnt from this exercise . . .

In the next chapter, we will help you take steps forward in getting out of your head so that you can enjoy more of your social life.

Key points and giving yourself credit

 A huge well done for working through this chapter. You have made a big step forward today on the path to overcoming social anxiety. You might want to make a note of your key take-home points below.

If you found some of this tough, you are not alone – overcoming social anxiety is not easy, so give yourself a break. What would you say to a best friend or loved one if they had made a start by reading this chapter? Imagine you are sending them a message right now – what would you write? Maybe make a note of this and read it aloud to yourself. This is another step forward in starting to be a little kinder to yourself.

See Josh's example:

What I can give myself credit for	Key learning points
Reading through this chapter.	It makes sense why I feel so anxious.
Mapping my social anxiety cycle.	My anxiety is driven by my negative thoughts. I imagine I come across in a negative way and assume others see the same.
	Being so in my head (spotlight of attention on me) and doing the things I usually do (like preparing things to say) keeps it going.
Trying the exercise using and then dropping my self-focus and behaviour traps.	I feel better when not so focused on myself. I need to work on being more in the conversation and less in my head.

Now it's your turn:

What I can give myself credit for	Key learning points

Chapter 3

Getting out of My Head and Enjoying Social Situations

Elyse's reflections

I used to feel so self-conscious. I was so aware of myself that I couldn't connect with other people. Staying focused on myself was one of the biggest things that kept me stuck in my anxiety, as it meant I was constantly analysing every little thing I did. Getting out of my head was one of the most helpful things I did. Not only did I feel better, but it also gave me the chance to enjoy conversations.

In Chapter 2, we started to make sense of what is keeping you caught in the cycle of social anxiety. The 'Take action' exercise involved having a conversation. For the first few minutes you focused on yourself and then you switched it around and absorbed yourself in the chat. Like Josh, did you discover that you felt more anxious, more self-conscious when you focused on yourself? If you haven't had a go at the exercise yet, why don't you try now? It will give you an insight into the effects of being focused on yourself and help you on the path to feeling more confident.

Now, in this chapter, we will discover:

- Why being self-focused is unhelpful

- How you can get out of your head and start enjoying social situations more

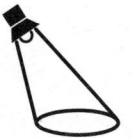

Do you feel under the spotlight when you feel anxious in social situations?

Do you become self-conscious?

Do you feel like you are the centre of attention?

When we feel anxious in social situations, our focus of attention turns inwards. We are focused on ourselves, on our feelings and how we think we look to other people. This can feel really uncomfortable.

For Nita, *In lessons, for example, when I am anxious, I get caught up in my head and I am really aware of feeling hot in my face, I am thinking about all the ways I am going to mess up, and I can picture how red and foolish I feel I look to everyone else. I feel so weird and different. I can hardly pay attention to what the teacher is saying.*

When we ask people **why** they become self-conscious when they feel anxious in social situations, most people tell us that they can't help it, it just happens. It is like a habit.

But if we wound the clock back, focusing on yourself probably started as a way of trying to work out how you come across to other people. If you were worried about coming across badly then it is understandable that you would watch and closely monitor yourself. But over time, it becomes automatic.

What is the problem with focusing on yourself? It makes you feel like you stand out.

Do you ever feel like the centre of attention? Or like you stand out from the crowd (and not in a good way)? When you're out and about, do you ever feel like you've got food on your face, or your skirt is hitched up, that there's something wrong with you and everyone is staring at you and making critical judgements about you?

Let's try to understand this feeling.

> *Josh was curious about it too. Why did he get this feeling of being stared at so strongly? What was going on? He decided to try an experiment to find out.*

Josh went out to his local shopping centre. He stopped and looked down at his feet for a few minutes. He focused his attention on himself and on how he thought he was coming across to passers-by. Josh noticed the familiar feeling of being stared at, of being judged by people. He was convinced that people were staring at him. So far, so typical.

But then, Josh did something different . . .

Josh looked up and around. He checked out the reality of whether people were staring at him. He looked around him like a hawk.

And he couldn't believe what he saw. No one was staring at him. People were looking ahead, looking down, looking at their phones, talking to one another. A couple of people glanced at him, but that was it. No one was staring at him. People didn't seem to look at him more than they looked at anyone else around him.

Josh was surprised. He tried the experiment a few more times. Every time, when he looked down, that old feeling of being stared at came back, but then when he checked it out the reality was very different and people were not staring at him.

So, what was going on? When Josh focused on himself, he felt he was being stared at. In other words, Josh was

> staring at himself. He was the centre of his own atten-
> tion. But he wasn't the centre of anyone else's.

Do you think this might explain what happens when you feel stared at too?

Don't take our word for it – try it out for yourself. It only takes a couple of minutes.

Take action

 Try out this exercise. Think of somewhere you can go where there will be quite a few people, such as a shopping centre, a park or bus stop.

When you get there, start by keeping your head down and avoiding eye contact with others. Bring on the feeling of being stared at by focusing your attention on yourself and on how you feel you are coming across to other people. You might notice this makes you feel anxious, but stick with it so you get the chance to learn something new.

Take a mental note of how many people you think are staring at you and how they are looking at you.

Then, look up and look around you. How does the reality compare to what you had pictured in your mind's eye?

Ask yourself: *How many people are staring at me?* If someone is looking at you, in what way are they looking? What are people doing?

Top Tips

★ Make sure you spend enough time *really* looking around you. Brief glances out of the corner of your eye aren't enough! Otherwise your imagination will fill in the gaps.

★ If you notice somebody glancing in your direction, try to keep their gaze for a moment to find out if they are staring at you or briefly parking their eyes in your direction. We all park our eyes briefly on people/cars/buildings we pass by – if we didn't we would constantly bump into each other. And we need somewhere to rest our eyes sometimes; it can get tiring constantly looking around. Often we choose to rest our eyes by 'parking' them on another person.

Here is a summary of Josh's experiment:

Step 1. Belief	Step 2. Situation	Step 3. Predict	Step 4. Do it!	Step 5. Reflect	Step 6. Look ahead
People stare at me.	Shopping centre.	Everyone will stare at me and look at me in an unfriendly way, as if I am weird. They will frown – 90%.	I will go to the shopping centre. Look down for a few minutes and focus my attention on myself, take stock of what I expect to see. Then look	I felt anxious when I was focused on myself, and I could feel people's eyes on me. But then when I looked up, no one was staring at me.	No one is staring at me. I am not the centre of anyone else's attention. I am the centre of my own attention. Feelings can be misleading.

up and look around to see what other people are doing.	People were looking ahead, looking down, looking at their phones, talking to one another. A couple of people glanced at me, but that was it. Re-rating of my original prediction: Everyone will stare at me – 30%.	I will try this when I'm walking around school and any other time I get this feeling of being stared at.

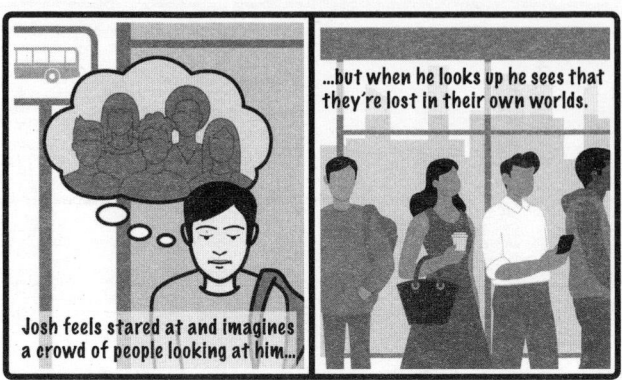

Josh was really staring at himself.
This gave him the illusion everyone else was too.

Why don't you give it a go? Let's test out the idea that when we are self-focused it can make us feel like everyone is staring at us, but it is actually just us staring at ourselves.

Step 1. Belief	Step 2. Situation	Step 3. Predict	Step 4. Do it!	Step 5. Reflect	Step 6. Look ahead
People stare at me.					

Taking it forward: whenever you feel stared at, use it as a cue to look up and check it out. It is a golden opportunity!

Elyse's reflections

If I was walking to school or was standing at the bus stop, I always felt like people were looking at me. Like I was standing in the way or standing in the wrong spot. In those moments I found it really awkward to look up at people to see if they were staring so I would start by trying to get lost in what was going on around me. Then I would scan around to see what others were doing – and realise that no one was looking at me. Nobody cares! They are minding their own business, busy living their own lives and having their own thoughts.

What is the problem with being self-focused? It makes you feel anxious.

The more you pay attention to anxious feelings, the stronger they feel.

When Nita is self-focused in social situations, she becomes hyper-aware of feeling flustered, shaky and hot, and then as she becomes more self-conscious about this, she feels even more of a weird nervous wreck and notices she gets more shaky and hot.

Take a moment to think about what happens to your anxiety feelings when you are self-focused in social situations. What do you notice about the effects of being self-focused on anx-ious feelings?

What is the problem with being self-focused? It triggers negative images and impressions of yourself.

Do you get images popping into your mind's eye of how you think you come across when you feel self-conscious? Do you come across like your worst fears realised? Nervous, anx-ious, the odd one out? Focusing on yourself triggers these images or impressions. We are going to learn more about these mental images and impressions in Chapter 4, Seeing Myself in a More Positive Way.

What is the problem with being self-focused? You miss out on what's going on around you.

When you're focused on solving a knotty problem or day-dreaming, you often miss what's going on in the here and now. That's because your head is elsewhere (with that maths problem or dreaming about the next holiday) and we only have a limited pot of attention to give to things at any one time.

In the same way, if most of our attention is taken up with ourselves and worrying about how we are coming across then there won't be much left to give to what is going on around us.

The problem with this is that we won't be able to spot how people are reacting to us in the moment. If you aren't focusing on other people, then you won't notice signs that they are interested in you or that they aren't reacting to you like you feared.

So when we are self-focused, we don't get the chance to 'reality test' our fears, because we aren't paying attention to the evidence we are getting. We just play the same old loop of self-critical thoughts in our head.

You might also notice that, when you are lost in your head, it can be hard to follow what others are saying. As a result, it can be even more difficult to stay involved in the conversation.

What were you focused on at the time? You were probably lost in the moment, absorbed in the here and now of what you were doing.

Remember back to a time when you really enjoyed listening to music, dancing or exercising. What were you thinking about at the time? Most likely, the answer is nothing! You were lost in the moment, absorbed in the here and now of what you were doing.

And that is the other problem with being self-focused in social situations. It makes it really hard to be in the moment, lost in the flow of it, and to have fun.

Think back to your favourite times with family or close friends. What were you focused on then? Nothing, right?!

Just the moment. To fully enjoy social situations we need to get out of our head and into the world.

> **Getting out of our heads and into the world is one of the keys to unlocking our social confidence.**

Take action

 So how can we get out of our heads and into the world? These exercises will help strengthen your attention muscle and help you to get lost in the moment when you're in social situations. So let's go to the attention gym and start practising getting out of your head.

Because being self-focused has become a habit, it takes a little practice to get used to being focused on what is going on around you in the outside world (being 'externally focused'). The good news is that we have five quick and easy exercises that you can do right now, from the comfort of your own chair, to help you get out of your head and into the world.

Let's begin.

Exercise 1. Sounds around

Where are you reading this? For the next couple of minutes, put the book down, shut your eyes and listen to the sounds you can hear around you. Really listen.

The radiator, the traffic, an aeroplane, birdsong, children playing, doors closing, the sound of a fridge . . .

Count as many sounds as you can – try to get to ten if you can. Pause on each sound – how near or far is it? What is it like? Is it clear or muffled? Is it constant or does it come and go? Focus as intently as you can on the sounds around you. If you find yourself caught up with a thought or worry, bring yourself back to a sound.

Now that you have spent some time listening to the sounds around you, take a moment to reflect on what it was like.

How did you find that? Most people tend to feel calmer and less tense when they are focused on the sounds, and more connected and involved with the world around them. Was that your experience too? It can be helpful to try it a couple of times.

Well done on making a start! It might not have felt like much, but this is a great first step to getting out of your head.

Exercise 2. Colours

This time we are going to try an exercise with our eyes open. For the next few minutes, put this book down and look around you and absorb yourself in the **colours** you can see around you. Don't look at objects and things but notice the different colours and the shades of those colours. Really look.

Pastel shades, primary colours, greys/reds, different shades of greys/reds . . .

Try to lose yourself in the colours around you. If you become distracted by a thought or worry, bring yourself back to a colour or shade.

Look for the colours of the rainbow around you. Red, orange, yellow, green, blue, indigo, violet. How many colours can you see?

Now that you have spent some time looking at the colours around you, take a moment to reflect on what it was like. Did you notice more than you might normally? Did you notice yourself feeling a little less tense? People tend to feel more connected with their environment and less tense when they try out this exercise. You might like to try it a couple of times.

Exercise 3. Light and shade

Now for something a little different. This is an exercise with your eyes open. For the next few minutes, put this book down and look around you and absorb yourself in how the light falls around you. Don't look at objects and things but notice where it is light and dark around you, how the light falls, where it is darkest, what are the shadows cast by different objects. Really look.

Try to lose yourself in the pattern of light and shadow around you. If you become distracted by a thought or worry, bring yourself back to the light and shadow.

Exercise 4. Sound switching

We are returning to a focus on sounds now, but this time we're going to listen to a piece of music. Grab your phone, pop your headphones on or earbuds in and choose a piece of music to listen to. Perhaps one you haven't heard for a little while. Now, as you listen to the music, select a particular instrument to focus on. You could try starting with a focus on the vocals, then moving to the percussion, then the keyboard . . .

What did you notice when you tried listening to the music this way?

Exercise 5. Talking

Pull up a video of someone chatting to camera, for example a video of your favourite influencer or celebrity. While watching it, really focus your attention on the person on screen – on what you find interesting about them and what they are saying. You could try switching your attention from focusing on the video for a few minutes to then focusing in on yourself, and then back onto the video.

Elyse's reflections

For me, practising with music was my favourite way to get out of my head, because I love blasting my music. If you can keep up some practice, even just five minutes every day, making an effort to consciously focus your attention elsewhere, out of your head, it helps you stop the spiral of anxious thoughts. I found that spending a few minutes getting lost in some music or looking out of the window and focusing on what I could see, helped me get out of my head and re-evaluate things.

When I got out of my head, I felt more connected to the world around me and it felt relaxing and safe.

Picking something you enjoy to help with getting out of your head is going to make it so much easier. For me that was music. For you it might be art – so getting lost in the colours around you.

Take-home messages from the exercises

What did you notice from these exercises? How did it feel when you focused on the sounds or sights around you? How did the world seem?

This is what young people have told us about their experience of getting out of their head:

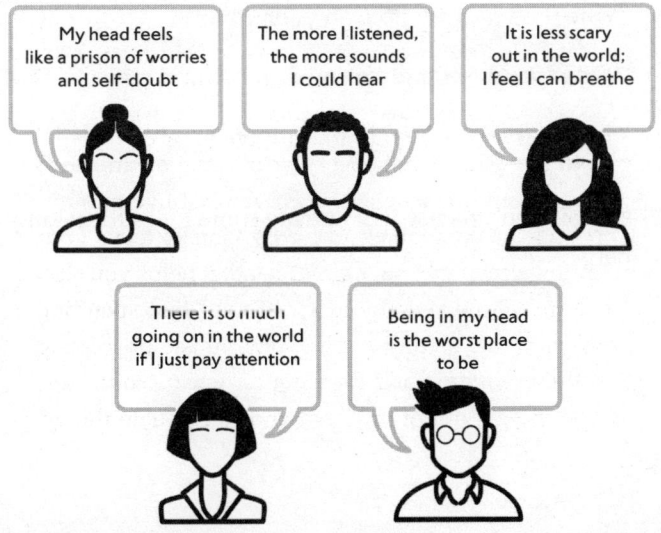

How would you summarise what you discovered from trying out these exercises?

Remember it takes practice to get used to being externally focused. Aim to practise every day if you can. Little and often is a good rule of thumb.

How can you remember to do it for a few minutes every day?

You could:

- Put a reminder on your phone

- Write it on a sticky note on your wall

- Ask a friend or family member to remind you

- Practise it *with* a friend or family member

Where can you practise it? Here are some ideas for taking it further:

➜ Class

Lessons in college or school are a golden opportunity to practise being externally focused. Really focus on what is being discussed, what the teacher is saying. Focus on what you find interesting about the lesson.

➜ Journeys

When you are travelling somewhere, like walking to school or driving to visit family, use this as an opportunity to absorb yourself in the sounds or sights around you.

➜ Trips

Try these exercises when you go to an art gallery, concert or the movies.

➜ Listening to music

When you are at home listening to music, keep trying out moving between the different instruments.

➜ Conversations

Why don't you practise being externally focused when you are with other people? Remember that it will feel more difficult to be externally focused in social interactions, because you are likely to be particularly self-conscious in these moments. As much as you can, tune in to what the other person is saying. If you spot yourself becoming self-conscious, try to redirect your attention back to what you can see and hear.

➜ Anywhere and everywhere

You can try cueing into sounds or sights wherever you are, whatever you are doing. Practising little and often is the key!

Key points and giving yourself credit

 Reminder! Don't forget to give yourself credit every time you have a go. Sometimes practice will feel easier than at other times; this is to be expected, but it is great that you have tried. And you will probably find that you like some of the exercises more than others, which is no problem; just keep up the practice and get strong at being externally focused.

See what Josh wrote:

What I can give myself credit for	Key learning points
I found it really hard to remember to do the practice. I noticed after a few days I hadn't done it at all. So, I decided to start with my walk to school. I put a reminder in my phone for when I left the house. I managed to get into the habit of doing it most days.	It was worth pushing myself to practise. My walk to school used to be full of worry about seeing people from school on the way and worry about the day ahead. I liked focusing on the sounds around me most. It made me feel calm and steady. I got to school in a much better place.
I find I get really self-conscious in class, and I was worried about trying to get externally focused in lessons. But I decided to try it out.	This was an eye opener. Focusing on what the teacher was saying and the lesson meant I felt less stressed and I picked up much more of the topic as well. Usually I'd spend the evening trying to catch up on the lesson topics, but now I feel more up to speed with them.

Now it's your turn:

What I can give myself credit for	Key learning points

Chapter 4

Seeing Myself in a More Positive Way

'I look like an idiot'

'I come across so dull'

'I see myself looking so red'

'I just look like a nervous mess'

You are most likely reading this book because you are concerned that you come across badly to others. But unlike the star of a reality show, who is followed by a camera crew all day, you probably don't see your chats played back. When we are struggling with social anxiety, we can feel convinced that we come across badly. But in truth it is physically impossible to see ourselves through the eyes of others. So in the following pages we are going to find out:

- How we know how we come across

- Where we get our ideas about this from

- How accurate these ideas really are

The way you see yourself is key

Did you know that the way you picture yourself in your mind can have a big impact on how you feel? In a study done at our clinic, when young people with social anxiety were asked to picture themselves looking anxious during a conversation, their anxiety levels jumped up, compared to when they pictured themselves looking relaxed.

Is it a fact or a feeling?

At the start of this book, we looked at how you see yourself in social situations. Look back at the notes you made in your map of social anxiety. If you didn't write anything, take a moment now to cast your mind back to the last time you felt anxious about how you were coming across. It may help to ask yourself:

- How did you picture yourself looking? Did you have an impression of what others might see?

- If an artist was drawing a picture of you at this moment, what exactly would you tell them to draw?

Make a few notes below about what your self-image or impression looks like.

What was giving you the idea you were coming over in this negative way? Did you ask others how you were coming across? Were others saying this is how you looked? Or was it how you imagined you looked when you were feeling self-conscious?

We know from research that when people are feeling socially anxious they tend to zoom in on themselves and how they are feeling. If we feel anxious inside our body, we tend to build a picture of ourselves looking anxious to others based on this. But feelings can be misleading. We often don't look how we feel.

Nita felt she looked red and shaky when around others. On one occasion she had once been told she looked hot, but she had little evidence that this is how she looked most of the time. Nita was using her anxious feelings, and her memory of this one time, to guide how she thought she looked to others most days.

Elyse's reflections

I had a very negative self-image. I was conscious of my eye contact when speaking to other people. I would start blinking and focusing on my facial muscles. They felt twitchy to me. Then I imagined that I was coming across in an unusual way to other people. It was like I could see myself through the way my muscles felt. I imagined I looked twitchy, even though I didn't physically look that way.

Are feelings noticeable on the outside?

What goes on inside our body is mostly hidden to other people. Think about when you feel really hungry. You might feel strong hunger pangs that are hard to ignore, but this feeling would be largely invisible to others. Even the odd growl of your stomach would sound much louder to you than it would to anybody else. Our anxious feelings are the same. They are private, noticeable to you, but mostly hidden from others. Earlier in this book we compared this to listening to music through headphones. You might hear your favourite tune through your headphones, even feel the base vibrating through your body, but others can't.

We may feel like the moment our anxiety steps up a notch it changes how we appear, but does it? Take a look below at a young woman giving a talk at college. In the picture on the left she feels pretty calm. In the picture on the right, as she starts her talk, her anxiety leaps up. But as an outside observer, do you notice a big difference between the two images? Would you say she looks much more anxious when she stands up? Are her feelings as noticeable on the outside as she feels they are?

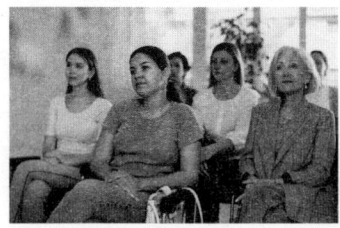 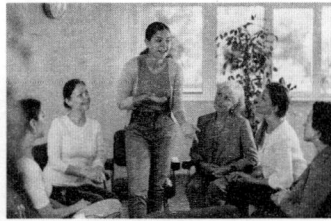

Does this young woman look much more anxious
before she gives her talk (picture on the left) or when
she gives her talk (picture on the right)?

The young woman **feels** more anxious when she stands up and so she jumps to the conclusion that she looks anxious. But these are feelings, not facts.

What does the camera show us?

In a study done at our Oxford University clinic, people having treatment for social anxiety were video recorded having a conversation with somebody they had not met before. Before viewing the video of the conversation, they thought they would look pretty anxious. When they watched themselves back, they saw they came across much better. They didn't look nearly as anxious as they felt – their feelings had deceived them. You can see this in the graph below.

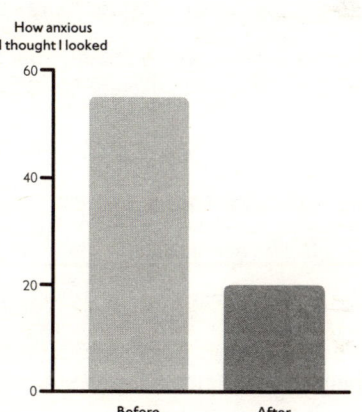

How anxious people thought they looked before and after watching themselves on video

So if our feelings are a terrible guide as to how we are coming across, we need to start focusing more on the facts – and we will show you how.

Become a fact (not a feeling) detective

Nita was starting to realise that she had been relying on her feelings to guide how she thought she looked. She was wondering how reliable her feelings really were. Nita had struggled with social anxiety for the last four years and had felt anxious at some point on most of those days. She used her phone to calculate that this was around 1,460 times she had felt anxious around others (once a day x 365 days in a year x 4 years having social anxiety). Nita considered how many of those times she had hard evidence that she came across as red and shaky. Although she had felt this way multiple times, she could only think of one occasion when others had commented that she looked hot. She decided that instead of just going on how anxious she felt, she needed to start to hunt for the facts about how she came across.

If you have a negative image or impression of how you come across you are not alone. Be kind to yourself. It can be hard to see yourself in such a negative way. The good news is that by becoming a fact detective rather than focusing on our feelings, we can change the way we see ourselves and this can help us feel more socially comfortable.

Would it be OK for a police officer to arrest somebody without any evidence because they **felt** they were guilty? No!

Feelings are not good evidence. So we need to get a little better at looking for evidence and not using our feelings to judge how we see ourselves.

Here are four exercises to help you do this:

Take action

Exercise 1: Become a reality show star (for the sake of this exercise only!)

 Let's begin with a short exercise to help you to practise focusing more on the facts, rather than on your feelings. We are going to try to picture a recent social situation through the view of a camera, seeing only what is visible on the outside.

Think about a recent time when you **felt** socially anxious and as if you came across in a negative way. Write out briefly what happened in the box below, and try to include:

- How you were feeling

- How you saw yourself in your own mind

- What happened next

- How others actually responded to you (i.e. what they did or said)

This is what Nita wrote:

I was talking to a group of girls after a class and some-body asked me a question. I felt really hot in the face and imagined I looked really red. My hands felt shaky and my heart was racing. I thought I looked really anxious and foolish. I changed the topic of conversation and somebody else started talking about where to go for lunch. We then went to the canteen.

Now, let's imagine that you are the star of a reality show and you have a camera crew following you. OK, this might be your worst nightmare, it is certainly ours, but stick with us for the sake of this exercise! Let's imagine you have the footage of the situation above captured on camera. Read over what you wrote above and then cross out anything that would **not** be picked up by the camera.

- Cross out anything you felt inside your body that the camera wouldn't see, e.g. feeling sweaty, feeling red, feeling shaky, feeling anxious

- Cross out any private thoughts you had about how you looked, e.g., *I think I look foolish*

- Leave only factual evidence in the account, e.g. how others responded and what happened next

Here is Nita's account after she has crossed out anything that a camera would not see (her thoughts and feelings), leaving only the facts:

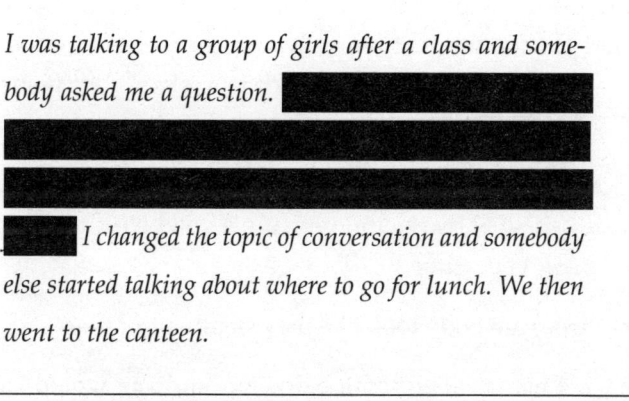

I was talking to a group of girls after a class and some-body asked me a question. ▓▓▓▓▓▓▓▓▓▓▓
▓▓▓▓▓▓▓▓▓▓▓▓▓▓▓▓▓▓▓▓▓▓▓▓▓
▓▓▓▓▓▓▓▓▓▓▓▓▓▓▓▓▓▓▓▓▓▓▓▓▓
▓▓▓▓ *I changed the topic of conversation and somebody else started talking about where to go for lunch. We then went to the canteen.*

Now read over your own account, considering that you have crossed out anything a camera would not see. What do you notice? If you only saw what the camera could see, would your sense of how you come across be more positive?

Take action

Exercise 2: Look at a photo

 You may not like looking at photos of yourself and might avoid doing this. You may even have seen photos or videos of yourself before and found yourself cringing. Let us reassure you – everybody does this! All people find it hard to watch themselves. This is because when we see ourselves our inner critic tends to pop up. We are much harder on ourselves than we are on others. But, if you can look at it without being hard on yourself, in the same way you would look at anybody else, looking at a photo or video of yourself can be a very powerful thing to do. Below we will show you how.

Are there any photos you can find of you in a group or the kind of situation that typically makes you feel anxious (e.g. at a family wedding, at a party or in a school class photo)?

If so, take a look at the photo – be sure to look at the whole group, not just yourself. Try to think of yourself in the photo as if it is somebody else, perhaps a good friend or a loved one. Ask yourself:

- Does anybody look like they stand out?

- If I was an alien coming down from space would I think that one of the humans looked significantly different or more anxious than the others in the photo?

- Do the other people in the photo look like they are responding negatively to you?

- How does the photo compare to the negative self-image you wrote out in this chapter?

- Try to ignore any self-critical thoughts – what would you say if it was your friend in the picture?

- Is it possible you look like an acceptable person, much like everybody else?

Make some notes about what you learnt:

Take action

Exercise 3: Take a video

 To get a more realistic image of how you come across in social situations it can help to look at a video of yourself.

You may already have some video of yourself you could look at. If not, you may want to ask somebody you trust to video you. Or you could try pretending you are giving a talk in class about a recent holiday you went on and stand up and record yourself speaking for sixty seconds on your phone or laptop.

Tip: If you do this, try saying whatever comes to mind without overthinking it.

Before you watch the video back, take a moment to write down how you felt you were coming across at the time. Write out the image or impression you have of yourself based on your feelings before viewing. For example Nita wrote, *I think I will look 80% trembly – you will see a noticeable shake and flustered – I won't make any sense.* Then try watching the video. Again, try to imagine you are watching a good friend or loved one speaking and ignore any self-critical thoughts. Ask yourself:

- Does that person look like they are really anxious?

- If I was an alien coming down from space would I think that person looked odd, weird or really anxious?

- How does the video compare to the negative self-image you wrote out in this chapter?

- Try to ignore any self-critical thoughts – what would you say if it was your friend in the video? What would be your overall sense of how they looked?

- Is it possible you look like an acceptable person, much like everybody else?

- Compare what you see on screen to how you predicted you would look based on your feelings. Is it possible you come across a little better than you felt you would?

Tip: If you find it hard to hear your own voice, try watching with the sound off for a few seconds first.

Nita wrote: *It was hard watching it back to start with, but when I turned the sound off and tried to imagine an alien watching the video, I realised I look like any other human. I wasn't as shaky as I predicted I would be and didn't look as flustered as I felt I would. I come across a bit better than I feel I do.*

Elyse's reflections

I really struggled with videoing myself and watching it back because of how embarrassing it felt. This is totally normal. You have to pretend that you don't know yourself and act as if you are looking at some random person talking and evaluate purely from what you see. I watched a conversation I had with somebody back on video and I realised what I was feeling didn't come across at all. It just looked like I was having a normal conversation. Seeing that really helped me put it into perspective. People aren't seeing what I'm feeling as much as I think they are.

Make some notes about what you learnt:

Take action

Exercise 4: Ask somebody you trust

 This may feel scary to do, but you could try asking somebody you trust (like a parent, sibling or close friend) about how they see you coming across when they speak to you. They won't have access to your feelings and so might be able to give you a more realistic picture of what others see.

Pulling it together and taking things forward

Thinking about everything you have learnt in this chapter and the exercises – what does this tell you about how you might come across to others? Is it possible your feelings aren't as visible as you thought they were? If so, it might help to write this down on a card or piece of paper or as a note on your phone. This is something you can look at to remind yourself of your more positive image the next time you are feeling anxious. You might find it helpful to put the card somewhere in your bedroom so that every time you read it you will be reminded of what you have learnt and it will start to sink in. You might like to put it on your bedside table, on your mirror, have it as a bookmark, or perhaps pop it face-up in your sock drawer. It doesn't matter where, as long as you will see it often and it feels comfortable for you. Remember – studies show that when we have a more positive image in our mind we feel less anxious – so the chances are this will help you feel more confident.

Below is Josh's card:

'I look less anxious than I think.

I look like a normal guy, smiling and chatting.'

What will you write on your card?

Once you've decided what you would like to write on your card, you can make it however you'd like. It could be by hand or computer: whatever works best for you.

Key points and giving yourself credit

 Give yourself credit for working on your self-image. You have made a great start in this chapter to try to look at yourself in a different way. As you move forward with this book you will discover other ways to find out how you actually come across, and your confidence will continue to grow.

See what Nita wrote:

What I can give myself credit for	Key learning points
Reading this chapter.	My feelings are not always visible.
Looking at a photo of myself with friends.	I was hard on myself at first, but when I imagined I was looking at somebody else I could see I came across much better than I felt I did.
Watching myself back on video.	
Asking somebody I trust.	I haven't asked somebody I trust yet, but I plan to speak to my best friend Jenny about it this week.

Now it's your turn:

What I can give myself credit for	Key learning points

Chapter 5

Letting the World Get to Know Me

'The world is flat!' – reality-testing our beliefs

Beliefs are like 'best guesses' about what is going on. We have information (what has happened in the past, what we have read, been told, what we can see and hear around us now) and we use this as a basis upon which to form our views.

That is why people used to believe the world was flat. Ships would sail off towards the horizon and often never return, so unsurprisingly people took this information and came to the belief that the world was flat.

It wasn't until curious scientists went out, asked questions and gathered data that this view was challenged. Scientists looked at the new information they had gathered and real-ised that the earth was, in fact, round. It seems obvious now, right? But it didn't at the time . . .

What has this got to do with building self-confidence?

It is about questioning, or reality-testing, our beliefs, whether these are beliefs about our planet or about ourselves.

In this chapter we are going to learn:

- How to reality-test our beliefs using confidence experiments

- The key steps for doing confidence experiments

- Top tips for getting the most out of confidence experiments

For now, let's spend a little longer thinking about why it might be important to reality-test our beliefs . . .

In Chapter 2, we talked about the thoughts you have when you feel anxious in social situations. Remember Nita, she thinks: *I'll mess this up, I'll get flustered, I'll look nervous and weird.*

These thoughts or beliefs are understandable. They're often based on things that have happened in the past, things people have told us. For example, after Nita had given a talk in her first year of secondary school, someone in her class blurted out, 'You look really hot.' Nita now remembered that every time she spoke in class, fearing she would blush and be humiliated. These types of thoughts can cause problems when they go unchecked.

Nita did the same thing every lesson. She was sure she was going to blush, stumble over her words and look nervous and weird. So, she focused on herself, looked down and kept as quiet as possible. And if the teacher did ask her a question, she would keep her eyes on her desk, rehearse what she was going to say in her head, and then speak as quietly and briefly as possible. It was like Nita was holding her breath until the class was over. Waiting for her next lesson, she was sure it would go wrong again, and so again in her next class, she would do the same things, hoping she would 'get away with it' this time as well. Nita didn't give herself the chance to discover that, in fact, she didn't blush or stumble over her words as she feared, and other people reacted to her just fine.

Does this sound familiar?

If my thoughts aren't facts, why do I still think this way?

It is no surprise that we all do things to try to prevent our fears from happening. We might hide our face if we are concerned about coming across as weird or looking nervous; we might keep quiet if we think we are boring; we might wear more layers if we are concerned about sweating so that we hide any possible wet patches. Many of these things can prevent us from reality-testing our fears. They can sometimes even cause some of the things we are worried about. You might remember we called these 'behaviour traps' earlier. Let's hear how Josh's behaviour traps kept his fears going.

Josh thought he was boring. When he met up with friends he kept quiet and asked himself, *How am I coming across?* He was often so in his own head he missed things the other

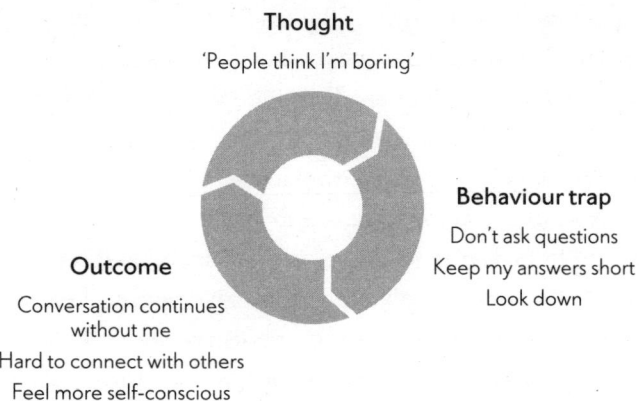

Thought

'People think I'm boring'

Behaviour trap

Don't ask questions
Keep my answers short
Look down

Outcome

Conversation continues
without me
Hard to connect with others
Feel more self-conscious

person was saying. He didn't really take part in the conversation. This made Josh feel more anxious and boring. It was also hard for others to get to know him, as he was so quiet all the time.

It is time to do things differently.

We are going to take a fresh look at our thoughts and fears and check out how they stack up in reality. We are going to be like the scientists who tested whether the world was round or flat. Let's not assume our fears are true, let's go and test them out.

And remember that the scientists went and tested their ideas out even though most people were sure the world was flat. But the scientists questioned the status quo. So even if you feel sure of your view of yourself, pretty certain you are going to mess up or embarrass yourself, why not try being curious, like a scientist? You might find out something interesting . . .

Nita decided to begin testing out her fears. Although she felt scared at the thought of it, she was interested to find out more about the reality of her fear that she would stumble over her words and people would laugh at her. She thought a good place to start would be in the classroom – the fear always seemed to pop up then and she was there every day! Nita took note of how certain she felt that her fears were going to come true – she thought about 80%. Then, when the teacher asked her a question, instead of rehearsing what she was going to say in her head and speaking as quietly and briefly as possible (her usual behaviour traps), she answered with what came to mind, spoke at her usual volume, looked up and around, and kept as focused on her teacher and classmates as possible.

Nita felt a tingle when she had done it. She was pleased with herself. No, proud of herself. This was challenging for her and it was a big step. But it was more than that. When she had answered the teacher's question, she found she could answer fine without all the usual rehearsal. In fact, it was easier to concentrate on the lesson and reflect on the topic when she was focused on it and not rehearsing things to say. And no one paid any particular attention to her. The lesson simply carried on. Her original predictions weren't right at all. Perhaps she could speak fine and come across OK as she is. Now that possibility was worth testing out a bit more . . .

The way to start testing out our thoughts is through **confidence experiments**.

The aim of confidence experiments is to test out our fears and discover what happens in reality. And the way to do this is by facing a situation we have been avoiding and make sure we follow the two golden rules of confidence experiments:

Golden rule 1: Drop our behaviour traps so we can discover what happens when we are not hiding away.

Golden rule 2: Get out of our heads so we can check out how people respond to us.

You might even have tried your first confidence experiment already. In Chapter 3, Getting Out of my Head and Enjoying Social Situations, we read about Josh's experiment to test out the feeling of being stared at. He did it by going to a shopping centre and following the two golden rules of confidence experiments. He looked up and around (**Golden rule 1**: Drop behaviour traps) and focused on what other people were doing (**Golden rule 2**: Get out of our heads). Did you try out the 'feeling stared at' experiment yourself? If you did, then congratulations, you have done your first confidence experiment already! If you haven't tried it yet, why don't you flip back to page 48 and take a look now? Lots of people find it a really good confidence experiment to start with.

You might have noticed that when Nita tested out her fears, she did things differently – she dropped her behaviour traps.

Here is another great confidence experiment to try out while you're getting going that can help you to discover the effect of behaviour traps. Let's hear from Nita what she did. For one of her first confidence experiments, she decided to test out the effect of behaviour traps. She planned to go and talk to a shop assistant in a shop (something she would usually avoid if she could). She planned to intentionally drop the behaviour traps – speaking quickly and quietly, hiding her face with her hair and avoiding eye contact. She planned to spot what happened to her anxiety and to her predictions.

She predicted: *I will go red and flustered and the shop assistant will get annoyed that I am taking up their time.* She felt pretty certain that this was going to happen (about 80% sure). To make sure she didn't use how hot and anxious she **felt** to judge the outcome, she thought about how the shop assistant might respond if they were annoyed. She predicted: *They will roll their eyes and be sharp with me.*

She went to a bookshop and approached a shop assistant. She asked them where a certain book was and she looked at the shop assistant, focused on what they were saying and let go of those behaviour traps.

OH! She felt much better than usual. She reflected on recent times when she had gone to the shops but had used her behaviour traps. This time, she noticed she could also speak more freely and concentrate on what the lady was telling her. She felt like this experiment really showed her how unhelpful behaviour traps are. She was glad she had done it. She was also pleased to see that the shop assistant didn't get annoyed and responded well.

Take action

 Why don't you try it out too?

- Pick a situation that makes you feel anxious, such as talking to a shop assistant

- Make a prediction about how they will react to you (focusing on reactions you can see and hear)

- Go to the situation, talk to the person while you **drop** your behaviour traps! You can go back and look at your list of behaviour traps in Chapter 2 if you would like a reminder

- Check out how they respond to you in reality

Here are the six steps to follow when doing confidence experiments:

The six steps of a confidence experiment

Step 1. Belief

What is one of the things you worry about a lot in social situations? If you are unsure what to choose, you could take a look at the answers you gave in Chapter 2 about negative thoughts.

Step 2. Situation

Think of a situation where you can test out your fear. It might be asking a question in class, chatting to your neighbour in class or ordering a drink in a café. A good rule of thumb is that any situation where you feel anxious or you have been avoiding or situations where you know you use a safety behaviour can be a springboard to a behavioural experiment. Think back, what are your goals? How do you want things to be different socially? Your goals can be another useful guide to where you might plan an experiment.

Step 3. Predict

Ask yourself: *What is the worst that you think might happen? How would I know that the worst had happened?*

Consider:

- What do I fear will happen? How do I fear I'll come across?
- What signs of anxiety do I fear I'll show (blushing, sweating)?
- How will I know that other people have noticed these things?
- What would be the worst thing about them noticing?

Rate how strongly you believe these will happen, from 0% (they won't happen) to 100% (they will definitely happen).

Step 4. Do it!

Remember the two golden rules of confidence experiments: drop our behaviour traps and get out of our heads so we can learn as much as possible from it.

Step 5. Reflect

Well done! Now take some time to compare what happened in reality to what you had feared. What does this tell you about your first fear? It can be helpful to re-rate your original prediction on a 0–100% scale.

And what does it tell you about how accept-able, how likeable you are as a person? Does it suggest you are more OK than you had thought? If you find it hard to come up with positive reflections about yourself then why don't you ask a trusted friend to help you, or answer the question as if you were answering for someone else?

Step 6. Look ahead

OK, now it's time to decide what experi-ment to do next. It could build on what you have just done. Sometimes we need to have another go, for example if we couldn't quite drop our behaviour traps the first time. We might want to test our fear out in a different way. Or it might be that it is time to test out a different fear.

It can be helpful to note down your confidence experiments – at both the planning and the reflection stages. We use a confidence experiment log to do this. The log looks like this:

Step 1. Belief	Step 2. Situation	Step 3. Predict	Step 4. Do it!	Step 5. Reflect	Step 6. Look ahead
What fearful belief will you focus on?	What situation will you test out your fear in?	What is the worst that you think that you might happen? How would you know? 0–100%	How will you test it out? Remember to get externally focused and drop behaviour traps.	What happened? Re-rate your prediction (0–100%). What does this tell you about yourself more generally?	What are you going to try next to build on your learning?

Remember Nita's experiment talking to a shop assistant? Here is the log she completed:

🐾 Step 1. Belief	🐾 Step 2. Situation	🐾 Step 3. Predict	🐾 Step 4. Do it!	🐾 Step 5. Reflect	🐾 Step 6. Look ahead
I blush and look anxious when I talk to strangers.	Go into a book shop and ask the shop assistant where a certain book is.	I will go red and flustered and the shop assistant will get annoyed that I am taking up their time. They will roll their eyes and be sharp with me – 80%.	Rather than speaking quickly and quietly, I will ask the shop assistant a question clearly and look at her without hiding my face with my hair or looking away. I will focus on how she responds to me and ignore my feelings.	I felt much better than I usually do. I could speak more freely and she didn't get annoyed with me or roll her eyes. I felt a little flushed and anxious at first but she didn't seem to notice or respond negatively. Maybe I come across a bit better than I thought I do.	I can try this out again a couple more times over the week when I go into other shops or cafés or by asking somebody for directions.

You might also remember Josh's 'feeling stared at' experiment? You can look back at the log he completed on page 50 for another example. You will find a blank confidence experiment log in the Resources section at the back of this book (page 356), you can download one from https://overcoming.co.uk/715/resources-to-download or, if you prefer, you can note them down on your phone. You might also like to add your experiments as you go along in this book. We know it is a real help to log your experiments somewhere – find the way that suits you best.

Confidence experiments for my fears

In the next chapter we take common fears one by one. But first, here are some useful pointers for you when planning and carrying out your own confidence experiments.

Top Tips

★ Do confidence experiments several times a week – the more the better

★ Confidence experiments can be quick, like making a cup of tea

★ Remember to make a clear prediction and follow the golden rules

★ Try to focus on how others actually respond, not on your feelings

★ Confidence experiments are the engine that will build your social confidence

Elyse's reflections

I recommend people start small. I think it's daunting to go into it with a very big experiment. For me, the idea of going into a shop and talking to a stranger felt impossible at first. It was very helpful for me to just start doing confidence experiments within my friendship group, or my family or people that I was comfortable with. That helped me build my confidence elsewhere and try with people I'm not as close with.

Nita started testing out her fears by doing confidence experiments, and she discovered that:

I had been hiding the real me for so long but then I started to test out my fears, by facing situations I found stressful while getting out of my head and dropping my behaviour traps. And it was amazing, I discovered that I come across just fine as I am, there is no need to hide or cover up!

Key points and giving yourself credit

 Well done for working through this chapter on confidence experiments. Take a moment to give yourself credit for any of the confidence tasks you tried. A great way to build on your learning and to start being kinder to yourself is to make some notes on what you can give yourself credit for and what you learnt from it.

Here is what Josh said:

What I can give myself credit for	Key learning points
I read the chapter.	Confidence experiments are the way to build confidence. The key is to face my fears and remember to drop my behaviour traps and get externally focused.
Planning confidence experiments.	I read over Chapter 2 to get ideas about what fears to tackle first. It can be hard to remember to do confidence experiments so I set myself reminders on my phone.
Carrying out and reflecting on my experiments.	My first few experiments were hard but I am really glad I did them. Because the experiments have shown me that I come across fine as I am. I don't need to hide away or put on an act. I am going to keep going with the experiments!

Now you have a go:

What I can give myself credit for	Key learning points

Chapter 6

Particular Fears

Back in Chapter 2, we asked you about the social fears that you experience, and you might have started testing these out using confidence experiments. In this chapter, we are going to focus in on the most common fears. You will find helpful information and tasks to build your confidence in each section. Please feel free to go to all the sections that are most relevant for you. If you find having conversations challenging, the sections on 'feeling boring', 'feeling stupid' and 'feeling like I'm unacceptable (weird – unlikeable – not good enough)' may well be helpful.

To get the most out of the sections, it can be a good idea to make notes and set yourself a reminder to try any tasks you can't do right away.

Feeling stared at

'Everyone's staring at me'

'People will stare at me'

Have you ever been walking in a busy place (e.g. heading to college or walking in the shopping centre) and felt like everybody was staring at you? Does it feel like you stand out from the crowd in some way? Feeling stared at can be a horrible feeling and a lot of people with social anxiety experience it. We covered this a little in Chapter 3, but as this is such a common fear we want to guide you through some steps to free yourself from it.

The feeling of being stared at is an illusion

The feeling of being stared at seems so real – but are people actually staring? Our research has found that people with social anxiety overestimate the number of people who are looking in their direction when they are feeling self-conscious. When we are super aware of ourselves it gives us the illusion that everybody else is too. **The problem is that we are staring at ourselves and we then feel like the world is too.**

Our behaviour traps keep the illusion going

When you feel stared at, do you tend to keep your head up and look around, watching others? Our guess is that in busy places you may do what most people do when they feel observed – you probably look down. But the problem is that when we look down we cannot see what is going on around us. All we have to go on is our feelings. As you may have discovered from the earlier chapters, our feelings are not a reliable guide to what is happening.

Can you see how others are really responding to you if you keep your head down?

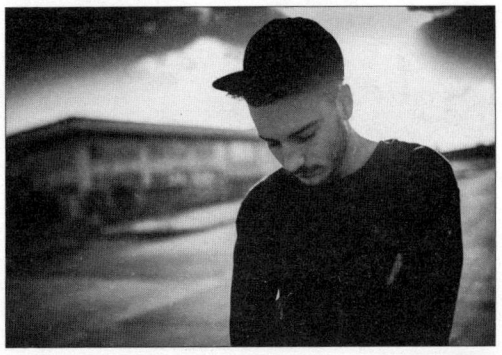

Below are some common behaviour traps we use when feeling stared at. Check if you use any of these and look at the ways they may be keeping you trapped:

Common behaviour traps we all use when we feel stared at

- Keep my head down
- Avoid eye contact with others
- Wear a cap or headphones
- Avoid going to busy places
- Avoid going to busy places alone
- If I do look up, I only take quick glances at what is going on around me

Others:

Ways they may be keeping me trapped

Without our awareness, these can:

- Make me feel more self-conscious
- Make it impossible for me to find out if people are looking at me or how they are reacting
- Make me feel more anxious
- Stop me doing things I want to
- Lead to me feeling weird, different or odd

Others:

Take action

Tasks to build your confidence in public

The staring experiment

 We have a neat confidence experiment to help you put the illusion of feeling stared at to the test.

We already suggested this task in Chapter 3, but if you haven't tried it, or still feel like others stare at you, we recommend you give it a go. Here are the steps to follow:

Step 1: Think of somewhere you can go where there will be quite a few people, such as a shopping centre, a park or bus stop.

Step 2: When you get there, start by keeping your head down and avoiding eye contact with others. Bring on the feeling of being stared at by really focusing your attention on yourself and how you feel you are coming across to other people. You might notice you feel uncomfortable, but try to stick with it so you get the chance to learn something new. Make a mental note of how many people you think are staring at you and how they are looking at you.

Step 3: Then look up and look around you. How does the reality compare to your prediction? Ask yourself: *How many people are staring at me?* If someone is looking at you, in what way are they looking? What are people doing? What are they actually focused on?

Trouble shooting: If you notice that one or two people look in your direction, try not to look immediately down or away.

Instead, keep their gaze for a second or two to see what happens. What you will most likely discover is that the person was not staring at you, or thinking anything negative about you, but that they were simply parking their eyes on you before they move on to the next person/object/building to look at.

You may want to make a note of what you discovered:

WHAT IS EYE PARKING?

You may occasionally notice that people do look in your direction. This is normal and does not mean that you are being stared at. It is called 'eye parking' (you might remember we talked about this in Chapter 3, see page 49).We must look at something when we walk down the street. Sometimes we look at cars, sometimes buildings or trees, sometimes people. If we didn't park our eyes on things briefly, what do you think would happen? We would all collide into each other! How many people have you glanced at over the years? Can you remember them all? Were you thinking anything about them at the time? Our guess is the answer to this is no! So, the next time somebody parks their eyes on you, don't assume they are staring because you stand out negatively.

Build your confidence by glancing back. What you will probably discover is that they soon park their eyes on something else. It is just what people do.

Elyse's reflections

If people glance at you, it's just a normal reaction to glance at movement and your surroundings. It's an instinct, and then they'll look away because it's not interesting enough to keep paying attention to. The staring experiment really helped me. If you can do it, it is some of the strongest evidence you'll ever get that people don't care as much as you think they do. It can feel tough to do it but the pay-off is worth it.

STARING – IS IT ALL BAD?

Hopefully, from trying the staring experiment you will have discovered that the feeling of being stared at is an illusion. That the only person really staring at you is yourself. But even if you do notice somebody looking for longer in your direction – it doesn't always mean they are thinking something about you at all. They may be thinking about their homework, their lunch, a falling-out with a friend. If they are giving you a second thought, could it even be a positive one?

Take a moment to think about things/people that you look at for longer than you usually would. If somebody catches your eye on the street – are you always thinking something bad about them? We have surveyed people about this, asking them what might make them look at somebody else for longer than usual. The kind of responses we got included:

- I might glance for longer at somebody if I like what they are wearing

- If I'm daydreaming about something else and I don't realise I'm looking at somebody

- I found myself drawn to looking at somebody the other day because I liked their hair colour

- If I'm bored on the train I might look around more at people, but I'm usually focused on what music I'm listening to and not thinking much about other people

- I might look at somebody if there was something I liked about them or found interesting, e.g. reading a book or comic I also like

Become a people detective!

In the coming days we suggest you think of yourself as a detective. Your mission is to observe others rather than yourself. What are they up to? What are they focused on? What do people do when they are out and about? How many people are looking at their phones? How many are wearing headphones? Is anybody reading? Becoming a people detective is a great way to help you keep your head up and your eyes off the floor. Instead of focusing on yourself, get lost in the world around you. Hopefully you will keep gathering data that other people are not as focused on you as you thought. Most people are caught up in their own world. They are focused on what they are doing, where they are going, the day-to-day of their own lives.

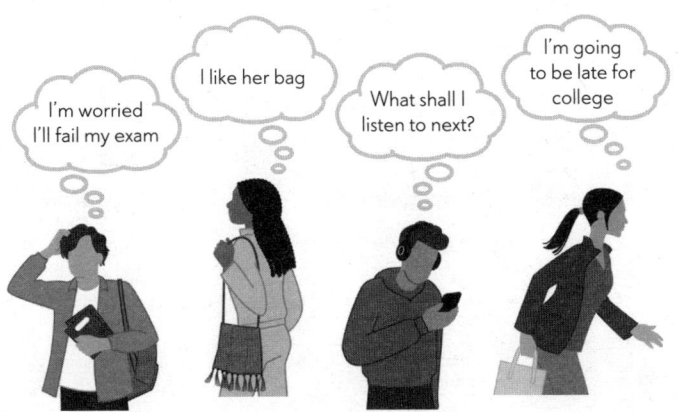

People are not staring at you. You look like any other acceptable person walking down the street. You do not stand out in a negative way.

Feeling stared at is a golden opportunity

There might be days when we are feeling more self-conscious than at other times, and the feeling of being stared at comes back. Let's say you have a spot right in the middle of your face that just won't go down or you've just changed your hairstyle. At these times we might be more inclined to look down in busy places. Instead, we need to use the feeling that we are being stared at as a golden opportunity to look up and test it out. Nita tried doing this for a week. Take a look at her confidence log below. The more Nita put her fear of being stared at to the test, the more her fear reduced.

Step 1. Belief	Step 2. Situation	Step 3. Predict	Step 4. Do it!	Step 5. Reflect	Step 6. Look ahead
What fearful belief will you focus on?	*What situation will you test out your fear in?*	*What is the worst that you think might happen?* *How would you know?* 0–100%	*How will you test it out?* *Remember to get externally focused and drop behaviour traps.*	*What happened?* *Re-rate your prediction (0–100%).* *What does this tell you about yourself more generally?*	*What are you going to try next to build on your learning?*
Feeling stared at.	Public busy places – whenever I feel stared at.	I often felt like 80% of people stare at me and give me weird looks.	Over the week, whenever I feel stared at I will make a prediction of how many people I FEEL are staring and then look up and around and find out	Monday: Walking into the exam hall felt like 80% of people were staring but most people were focused on their papers. Tuesday: In a café with Mum	I'll keep this up by observing others as much as I can over the week – walking with my head up rather than looking down when in busy places.

what people were doing.

eating an ice cream and felt like people were watching me eat, but looked around and they were talking or on their phones. 0% staring.

Wednesday:
Walking to shops, felt stared at but when I looked up only one person glanced and then looked away.

Maybe I don't stand out in a weird way; I'm like any other girl walking down the street.

Re-rated prediction:

People are staring at me – 30%.

Now it's your turn:

Step 1. Belief	Step 2. Situation	Step 3. Predict	Step 4. Do it!	Step 5. Reflect	Step 6. Look ahead
What fearful belief will you focus on?	What situation will you test out your fear in?	What is the worst that you think might happen? How would you know? 0–100%	How will you test it out? Remember to get externally focused and drop behaviour traps.	What happened? Re-rate your prediction (0–100%). What does this tell you about yourself more generally?	What are you going to try next to build on your learning?

Key points and giving yourself credit

 Well done for working through this section on feeling stared at. It is not easy to face your fears. Pause now and give yourself some credit for any of the tasks you tried. This is a chance to try being kinder to yourself and to build on your learning.

For example, Nita wrote:

What I can give myself credit for	Key learning points: Feeling stared at
Reading through the section on feeling stared at.	• Feeling stared at is a common fear but it is an illusion! • The feeling comes from staring at myself. • People with social anxiety overestimate how many people are staring at them. • Looking down when I feel stared at keeps me stuck. • People do park their eyes on things (I do too!), but it doesn't mean they are staring or thinking anything negative about the things they look at.
My confidence tasks: The staring experiment.	• This was powerful – nobody was staring at me! My feelings are not reliable.

Being a person detective.	• People are mostly on their phones, in their own world, talking to others. Not zoomed in on me.
Use feeling stared at as a golden opportunity.	• I found that whenever I felt stared at and I looked up and around, mostly people weren't staring at me. I don't stand out in a negative way.

Now it's your turn:

What I can give myself credit for	Key learning points: Feeling stared at

Feeling boring

'I'm boring'

'Others think I'm boring'

What is boring anyway?

It might surprise you to know that many people worry about others thinking they are 'boring'. But what does it mean to be boring? When you meet up with friends are you thinking: *I hope everybody fascinates me tonight,* or, *If I don't find every comment interesting, I want nothing more to do with these people?* We imagine not!

Conversations are not a performance

Do you feel like you need to perform in a social situation? If so, you aren't alone. Lots of socially anxious young people see social situations as a performance, something they need to do well at. But this puts a huge amount of pressure on you. In reality others aren't rating our performance on a 0–100% scale. They aren't turning up thinking, *I really hope Josh performs well tonight and gives me an interesting time.* You may **feel** like you need to perform around others, but in fact most social chat is about sharing the ins and outs of our day-to-day lives: what we watched last night; what we have for lunch; how annoying our parents are; what homework we have. Sharing the small things is an important part of feeling connected. If every conversation was 100% fascinating it would be a brain overload.

Take action

Find out for yourself

 **How fascinating are conversations really?** The next time you are on the bus or waiting in line, listen to the chatter around. You might be surprised to hear people simply sharing the ins and outs of their day-to-day lives. Most conversations aren't fascinating, they aren't a performance. Mostly socialising is simply about hanging out – sharing the same space.

You might want to take note of all the times you see people saying the kinds of things you might worry are boring and how the people they are speaking to react. For example, Josh worried that if he spoke about a topic that wasn't fascinating at some length others would think he was dull and not want to talk to him again. He spent a week looking out for times other people did the exact things he worried about and observed what others did. This is what he found:

Times I notice others talking about less fascinating topics	How others responded
Jake was talking about homework on Friday.	Everybody joined in and then the topic moved on. People still wanted to talk to him. They didn't react as if they thought he was boring.
In the lunch line I heard somebody talking a lot about the long drive they had to take on holiday.	Her friends listened and moaned about their own holiday. Nobody rejected her.
Amar was talking about Sports Day for a long time in break.	The others didn't seem to mind. They all spoke back and then the chat moved on.

Now it's your turn:

Take action

Make some notes about what you noticed here or in your notebook/on your phone.

Times I notice others talking about less fascinating topics	How others responded

What traps us into feeling boring?

When we worry we are coming across as boring we tend to put the spotlight of our attention onto ourselves. This back-fires and can instantly make us feel more boring. There are also common behaviour traps that we can fall into when we worry we are boring. Take a look at the table below which shows some common ones. Ask yourself, *Without realising it, could any of these keep me trapped feeling boring? Could they have a knock-on effect on my relationships?*

For example, Josh realised that by keeping quiet he was feel-ing more boring. He also thought that this might be giving other people the message he wasn't interested in talking to them, when the opposite was true.

Some of us may try too hard to come across well, e.g. making jokes or trying to sound interesting. This is stressful as it puts us under a lot of pressure. Putting on a front also stops us feeling accepted as we are.

Common behaviour traps we all use when we feel boring

- Keep quiet
- Stay on the edge
- Avoid groups or social occasions
- Head down
- Monitor how boring I am
- Think of interesting things to say
- Rehearse my sentences
- Try to come across well
- Try to entertain others (jokes, etc.)
- Compare myself to others
- Pretend I'm busy on my phone
- Focus on myself not others

Others:

Ways they may be keeping me trapped

Without our awareness, these can:

- Make me feel more boring
- Make it hard for people to get to know me
- Make it hard for me to follow conversations
- Make it hard for me to think of things to say
- Mean I never feel accepted for who I am
- Mean I might come across as if I'm not interested in others

Others:

When we notice any side effects of our behaviour traps it is important to be kind to ourselves. Although what we are doing might not be as helpful as we thought, these behaviours are understandable given our fears. The important thing is that we can now do something about them.

'I'm boring': Reviewing the week with fresh eyes

Our self-critical thoughts and feelings are not the most reliable evidence of how we are coming across. We would like you to consider the last week with fresh eyes. Rather than using your feelings to judge, are there any signs, however small, that others might not think you are boring? Consider what you would spot if you were thinking about a good friend of yours and their last week. Are there any moments you would point out to them that show they are OK, any times when others accepted them?

Josh wrote things down like: *When I spoke to Jake about gaming he wanted to talk more about it. Invited to Mike's to watch the football.*

Any evidence over the week I am not as boring as I think and feel I am

If you find yourself thinking of a time you did feel boring, try asking yourself whether there could be another way of looking at that moment now with fresh eyes? Ignore your feelings and focus on the evidence. Could this have been your inner critic or your feelings deceiving you? Could this feeling have been driven by your behaviour traps at the time? If so, add these things to the table.

Josh added: *On the school trip, I started talking about the homework and felt boring. But looking at it with fresh eyes the others did end up chatting about it. Nobody acted as if they thought I was boring. I was probably feeling boring because I was too much in my own head.*

If you struggled with the above, be kind to yourself. It is hard to start to think about things differently. If you have a good friend or family member you trust, you might want to ask them to help you.

What would you say to a friend?

Imagine a friend of yours says the kind of thing you often worry other people would judge to be boring. Would you decide you didn't like them anymore? If somebody really rejected somebody else because they said something a bit boring, would that be someone worthy of respect? Would you want to be friends with somebody like that? Try to keep in mind that in your worst-case scenario – somebody rejects you because of something you say – this is most likely not somebody you would want to be friends with.

You are only one slice of a rather large pie

You may feel like you are 100% responsible for others feeling interested in a social situation and having a good time. But is this true? Think back to the last social situation you were in. What different things were impacting on your interest and enjoyment? There are lots of things that impact how much somebody will enjoy a social event. In addition to the people there, this can include:

❑   How well we are feeling

❑   Our mood at the time

❑   Our hormones

❑   Anything that happened earlier that day

❑   How tired we are

❑   If we are hungry

❑   If we like the place or activity

❑   The weather

If we were to imagine a pie chart that looked at all the factors that take some responsibility for our interest and enjoyment of a social event, each of these things would take a slice of the pie.

Josh often felt responsible for his mates feeling interested and enjoying the time when he met up with them. He realised he was feeling 100% responsible for his mates having a good time. He then tried to think of all the other things that had a role in how much fun people had and then drew this out in a pie chart. Below are the things he came up with:

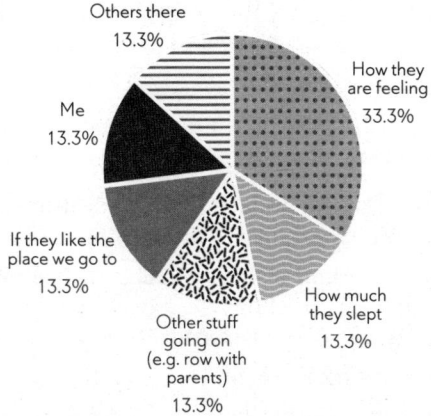

What things contribute to our enjoyment of a social event?

Others there 13.3%

How they are feeling 33.3%

Me 13.3%

If they like the place we go to 13.3%

Other stuff going on (e.g. row with parents) 13.3%

How much they slept 13.3%

If you find you take too much responsibility for others' enjoyment or interest, you might want to try writing down all the other things that also play a role. You could also draw your own pie chart out below, adding in these other things that contribute. Hopefully, you will see that you are one small part of the picture, a small slice of pie. After writing down all these things, Josh realised that his mates were also responsible for enjoying themselves; he didn't need to put so much pressure on himself to perform.

My pie chart

Take action

Confidence tasks to overcome feeling boring

1. Find out for yourself

 One of the most common traps we use when feeling boring is to monitor how interesting or not we think we are coming across. This back-fires and instantly makes us feel more boring.

To find this out for yourself, the next time you speak to some-body, start by asking yourself, *How interesting am I sounding?* Then monitor how boring you feel. After a short chat doing this, try things differently. Get out of your head and focus on the other person. Compare how each way of being in the conversation felt. You will most likely discover that you feel more boring when you are in your own head. The best way to feel more interesting is to get out of your head and get lost in the chat.

Elyse's reflections

I used to monitor myself a lot because I felt boring. So I tried a task where I didn't monitor myself, I just said what came to mind. It made me see that the feeling I was boring was really a component of me being very hard on myself and self-critical.

You might want to take some notes about what you noticed, below or in your notebook.

2. *Taking the pressure off yourself in conversations*

Some of us find that rather than being lost in the conversation we are too busy focusing on how interesting or not we are. This may mean we hold back and keep quiet or we try too hard to be the life and soul of the party, cracking jokes, not allowing any pauses in conversations. Either way, we are putting too much pressure on ourselves, and it is exhausting! It is time to take the pressure off yourself and go with the flow. Stop focusing on how interesting or not you are and instead get lost in the chat. If you find you try too hard to come across well, allow yourself just to be with others rather than trying to sparkle. Below is Josh's confidence experiment to take the pressure off himself. He tried this first with a close friend and then with other people over the week.

Step 1. Belief	Step 2. Situation	Step 3. Predict	Step 4. Do it!	Step 5. Reflect	Step 6. Look ahead
I'm boring.	After basketball – talking to my friend Tom.	If I don't plan things to say in advance, I won't have anything interesting to say and the others will think I'm boring, ignore me and leave – 70%.	Take the pressure off myself. Rather than focusing on how interesting or not I am and thinking of things to say, focus instead on Tom and the chat. Say whatever comes to mind without planning.	I was surprised to find I felt more relaxed when I focused on the chat rather than myself. I managed to say a few things without planning or overthinking and Tom didn't ignore me or leave.\n\nI enjoy things more when I take the pressure off myself.\n\nI'm boring – 40%.	I need to practise this more over the week with different people.\n\nThe more I can do this, the more confident I will feel, and the more I will believe that others don't think of me as boring.

The next time you talk to somebody, purposefully do something different. Instead of monitoring yourself, hiding away or trying to think of interesting things to say, be yourself, join in and say whatever comes to mind, without overthinking it.

You might want to start planning to do this in the next chat you are likely to have, but then keep it going in a number of conversations this week. The more you put the fears to the test, the more your confidence will grow.

Remember the two golden rules of confidence tasks:

Golden rule 1: Drop our behaviour traps so we can discover what happens when we are not hiding away.

Golden rule 2: Get out of our heads so we can check out how people respond to us.

Elyse's reflections

I used to talk a lot, just so that I would fill the space, to avoid pauses so people did not think I was boring. I tried a task of taking a step back. I allowed a pause and gave more space for the other person to speak. This really helped me build confidence in just letting the conversation flow by itself. I realised nobody thought I was boring when I took the pressure off and I was just myself.

Step 1. Belief	Step 2. Situation	Step 3. Predict	Step 4. Do it!	Step 5. Reflect	Step 6. Look ahead	
What fearful belief will you focus on?	What situation will you test out your fear in?	What is the worst that you think might happen? How would you know? 0–100%	How will you test it out? Remember to get externally focused and drop behaviour traps.	What happened? Re-rate your prediction (0–100%). What does this tell you about yourself more generally?	What are you going to try next to build on your learning?	

3. Letting others get to know me

As we discovered above, our behaviour traps stop others from getting to know us and keep our negative thoughts and fears going. So the best way to test our fears is to stop the traps that are keeping them going. If you tend to hide away, keep quiet or avoid saying much about yourself, it is time to share a little more of yourself. It is time to let others get to know you. This might mean speaking for a minute or two longer than you usually would, without monitoring how you are coming across.

Here is Josh's step-by-step plan:

Step 1. Belief	Step 2. Situation	Step 3. Predict	Step 4. Do it!	Step 5. Reflect	Step 6. Look ahead
I'm boring.	Chatting to friends at school on Tuesday.	If I talk a little more than I usually do I'll come across as boring – 60%. The others will ignore me, will push me out of the chat.	Observe them, talk more in the chat, don't monitor myself, say whatever comes to mind – don't plan interesting things to say.	It was hard at first but I tried to focus more on them than on myself. It was OK in the end. I said some things and they didn't ignore me or push me out. They chatted back. Maybe others think I'm OK. I now believe I came across as boring 20%.	I can keep going with trying this out in as many chats as I can in school over the week. Doing it more and more will build my confidence.

Now it's your turn:

Step 1. Belief	Step 2. Situation	Step 3. Predict	Step 4. Do it!	Step 5. Reflect	Step 6. Look ahead	
What fearful belief will you focus on?	*What situation will you test out your fear in?*	*What is the worst that you think might happen?* *How would you know?* *0–100%*	*How will you test it out?* *Remember to get externally focused and drop behaviour traps.*	*What happened?* *Re-rate your prediction (0–100%).* *What does this tell you about yourself more generally?*	*What are you going to try next to build on your learning?*	

4. Using feeling boring as a golden opportunity

The best way to stand up to your fear is to look out for any times that you feel you are coming across as boring and use these as a golden opportunity to drop your behaviour traps, focus on others and find out how they actually respond. Try to keep track of what happens by using a log like the one above or keeping notes on your phone.

Key points and giving yourself credit

 Well done for working through this section on feeling boring. It takes guts to face up to our fears. Pause now and give yourself credit for working on this fear and for any of the tasks you tried. Taking a moment to make a note of what you could give yourself credit for and what you learnt is a great way to practise being kinder to yourself and to build on your learning.

For example, Josh wrote:

What I can give myself credit for	Key learning points: Feeling boring
Reading through the section on feeling boring.	• Feeling boring is a common fear. • Chats are not a performance! • Focusing on myself and my behaviour traps is keeping me trapped feeling boring.
Trying the positive log.	• There is evidence in the week that others don't think I'm boring. I just often miss it.
My confidence tasks: Listening to others' conversations. Taking the pressure off myself in conversations. Sharing more of myself. Use the feeling that I'm boring as a golden opportunity to see how others respond.	• Most chat is sharing the day-to-day and is not always fascinating (e.g. about homework, lunch, etc.). • There are lots of factors that play a role in how much people enjoy social events – I am one small part. • I don't have to put on a front and try to come across well; I'm OK as I am. • Good friends accept me when I'm just myself.

Now it's your turn:

What I can give myself credit for	Key learning points: Feeling boring

Feeling stupid

'I'm stupid'   'Others think I'm an idiot'

Lots of people who feel socially anxious worry that they are stupid or that others will judge them to be stupid. You are not alone if this is one of your fears. The chances are you are much harder on yourself than you would be on somebody else. Think about the kinds of things that you think you do or say that make you stupid. If you saw anybody else saying or doing these things, do you think you would decide they were stupid? If not, why not? Could it be that you are much harder on yourself than you would be on anybody else?

How we get trapped feeling stupid

Some of us may fear coming across as stupid if we have previously been criticised, teased or put down by others for making a mistake. When we fear coming across as stupid we tend to watch ourselves closely – the spotlight of our attention falls onto ourselves. Putting ourselves under the spotlight means we focus on things that might go under our radar if it was anybody else. Zooming in on daily human errors we inevitably make (e.g. getting things wrong, not knowing the answer to everything) can make us feel more stupid. Some of our behaviour traps (like overly preparing) may mean it takes us more time to respond with the right answers to things, even though we know them. This can also make us feel stupid. Our behaviour traps can then keep us stuck feeling stupid. Take a look at the table below, which shows some common behaviour traps people use when they fear they are coming across as stupid. Which might you use? Think about how they might be keeping you trapped.

For example, Nita realised that she was always in her head trying to think of clever things to say that often she didn't say anything much at all.

Be kind to yourself – it is understandable why we may have started to do some of these things. We will help you to work on doing things differently, to escape your behaviour traps.

'I'm stupid': Reviewing the week with fresh eyes

The chances are you are being much harder on yourself than you would be on somebody else. We would like you to consider the last week with fresh eyes. Is there any evidence that you are not as stupid as you sometimes feel you are?

Nita wrote things down like: *I understood the geography homework when some others didn't. I had some ideas for the school play that got taken on board. I was talking to friends about shows and nobody said I was stupid.*

Have there been any times when **somebody else** did or said something that you would judge negatively if you did the same thing yourself? For example, did anybody else not know the answer to something or hesitate when asked a question? If so, what did you make of it? Did you immediately jump to the conclusion that they were stupid? Or did you think about it in a different way? Nita wrote: *Jenny said she didn't get the geography homework, but I didn't think much of it. This shows me nobody knows everything, and others won't always think I'm stupid if I don't know something.*

Common behaviour traps when we feel stupid	Ways they may be keeping me trapped
	Without our awareness, these can:
• Don't say much	• Make me feel more stupid
• Avoid talking about myself	• Make it hard for people to get to know me
• Don't share my opinion	• Make it hard for me to follow what is said
• Prepare things to say	• Mean that I miss key information in class
• Monitor if I'm coming across as stupid	• Make it hard to think of things to say
• Hold back	• Make me less likely to ask about things I don't know about, which can limit my learning
• Censor myself	• Mean I never feel accepted for who I am
• Rehearse my sentences	• Mean I might come across as distant
• Focus on myself, not others	
Others:	Others:

> **Any evidence over the week that I am not as stupid as I think and feel I am**
>
>

If you find yourself thinking of a time you did feel stupid, ask yourself if there is another way of looking at it with fresh eyes. Ignore your feelings and focus on the evidence. Could you have been too hard on yourself at this moment? Could this feeling have been driven by your behaviour traps at the time? If so, add these things to the table.

Nita added: *I didn't understand the instructions on Sports Day but then lots of us were confused about where to go, not just me.*

It is hard to start to think about things differently. Be kind to yourself if you found this tough. A good friend or family member whom you trust might be able to help you with this.

What would you say to a friend?

If you noticed a good friend said the kind of thing that you often worry people would think was stupid, would you decide you didn't want to know them anymore? If somebody really rejected somebody else because they made a mistake – would that be someone to respect or be mates with? Try to keep in mind that in your worst-case scenario – somebody rejects you because of something you say – this is unlikely to be somebody you would want in your life.

Take action

Confidence tasks to overcome feeling stupid

1. Find out for yourself: Observing others

 What kind of things do you worry you might say or do that others would judge as stupid? For example, Nita worried that if she said something irrelevant or if she didn't know the answer to something, others would think she was an idiot. To find out a bit more about this she decided to spend a week looking out for times when other people did the exact things she often worried about and observe how others responded at these times. Below are a couple of things she noted down.

Times I notice others saying 'I don't know' or saying something irrelevant	How others responded
Samir said he didn't know the answer in class on Wednesday.	The teacher just asked somebody else and people carried on. Not major news.
Alice started talking about a channel she subscribed to in the middle of a chat about music. It was a bit irrelevant.	It didn't seem to bother anybody. The chat moved on to what we have been watching. Nobody seemed to think she was stupid.
Jack didn't know a band that everybody else had heard of.	There was some banter about it, but then people moved on. Jack wasn't left out after; it wasn't such a big deal.

Try this yourself! Make a note of the kinds of things you worry about saying or doing and keep an eye out this week for times other people do these things. How do others respond when this happens? Hopefully what you will see is that we all make mistakes, nobody knows the answer to everything; this is part of being human.

2. Saying whatever comes to mind

The next time you talk to somebody, purposefully do something different. Instead of preparing things to say, monitoring yourself, hiding away or holding back, be yourself, join in and say whatever comes to mind, without overthinking it. Ignore that inner critic!

You might want to start planning to do this in the next chat you are likely to have, but then keep it going in a number of conversations this week. The more you put the fears to the test, the more your confidence will grow.

Here is Nita's step-by-step plan:

Step 1. Belief	Step 2. Situation	Step 3. Predict	Step 4. Do it!	Step 5. Reflect	Step 6. Look ahead
I'm stupid.	Doing group work.	If I speak up, I'll say something stupid and people will think I'm an idiot – 80%. The others will roll their eyes and laugh.	Say more during the group work without preparing in advance. Observe the others in the group. Don't focus on myself.	I managed to say a few things about the topic. Nobody laughed or rolled their eyes. The conversation just carried on. I might be more acceptable than I think. People think I'm an idiot – 30%.	I can try to take part more in all my classes this week without preparing what to say.

Now it's your turn:

Step 1. Belief	Step 2. Situation	Step 3. Predict	Step 4. Do it!	Step 5. Reflect	Step 6. Look ahead
What fearful belief will you focus on?	*What situation will you test out your fear in?*	*What is the worst that you think might happen?* *How would you know?* *0–100%*	*How will you test it out?* *Remember to get externally focused and drop behaviour traps.*	*What happened?* *Re-rate your prediction (0–100%).* *What does this tell you about yourself more generally?*	*What are you going to try next to build on your learning?*

The best way to stand up to your fear is to look out for any times that you feel you are coming across as stupid and use this as a guide to drop your behaviour traps, focus on others and find out how they actually respond.

3. Be human!: Saying 'I don't know'

None of us knows the answers to everything. In fact, the only way we learn is by asking questions and finding out more. If you fear you might come across as stupid you may avoid saying 'I don't know', which can limit how much you learn in life. Let's experiment with finding out what happens if we allow ourselves to be human and say, 'I don't know.'

Elyse's reflections

I had this idea that I had to get things right all the time, always know the answer, or others would think I was stupid. I now know, after my confidence task of asking a friend how to do the homework, that I'm not going to be thought of as stupid if I say I do not know something.

I was extra brave and asked my friend what they thought about the fact I did not know how to do the homework. When they responded like it was not a big deal this really helped it sink in for me. People are not as critical as I thought.

Step 1. Belief	Step 2. Situation	Step 3. Predict	Step 4. Do it!	Step 5. Reflect	Step 6. Look ahead
I'm stupid.	Chatting about homework with friends.	If I say I don't know how to do the homework, they will think I'm stupid – 60%. The others will roll their eyes, laugh and say I'm stupid.	Be honest, say I don't know how to do something. Observe the others and ignore how I feel – see how they react.	I did it! I said I didn't know how to do the homework. Nobody laughed or rolled their eyes. A couple of others said they didn't either. Jake did say he got it but seemed to enjoy explaining it to us. Re-rated prediction: Saying I don't know doesn't mean I'm stupid! – 30%.	I can try to be honest when I don't know the answers – others may not know either!

Now it's your turn:

Step 1. Belief	Step 2. Situation	Step 3. Predict	Step 4. Do it!	Step 5. Reflect	Step 6. Look ahead	
What fearful belief will you focus on?	*What situation will you test out your fear in?*	*What is the worst that you think might happen?* *How would you know?* *0–100%*	*How will you test it out?* *Remember to get externally focused and drop behaviour traps.*	*What happened?* *Re-rate your prediction (0–100%).* *What does this tell you about yourself more generally?*	*What are you going to try next to build on your learning?*	

Give yourself some credit

 Well done for working through this section on feeling stupid. Take a moment to give yourself credit for working on this fear and for any of the confidence tasks you tried. A great way to build on your learning and to start being kinder to yourself is to make some notes on what you can give yourself credit for and what you learnt from it.

Josh's example:

What I can give myself credit for	Key learning points: Feeling stupid
Reading through the section on feeling stupid.	• Feeling stupid is a common fear. • Focusing on myself and my behaviour traps are keeping me trapped feeling stupid.
Trying the positive log.	• There is evidence in the week that others don't think I'm stupid; I just often miss it.
Trying my confidence tasks: Listening to others' conversations. Trying the task of saying whatever comes to mind and dropping my behaviour traps. Being human and saying when I don't know something.	• Nobody knows everything. • It is human to make mistakes. • I am accepted when I say whatever comes to mind. • Most people think it's totally acceptable not to know everything – I'm only human! • We learn by saying 'I don't know'.

Now it's your turn:

What I can give myself credit for	Key learning points: Feeling stupid

Fear of blushing

'I'm blushing'

'Others will see me blush'

Do you feel yourself blushing at times? Congratulations – you are human! Much like we all have a heart that pumps blood around our body, humans all blush. Whether you are a prince, politician, singer, actor, student, it doesn't matter – it is a bodily function. When blood rushes to our cheeks, how we think it looks might vary from person to person depending on our skin tone. Some of us may feel as though we flush red when we blush. If we have a darker skin tone we might feel as though our skin glows or shines in a noticeable way. But if we all blush at times, why do some of us worry about blushing more than others?

What does a blush mean to you?

The secret is in the meaning we apply to blushing. Those people who worry less about blushing tend to brush it off as something that happens to everybody at times. Those of us who fear blushing tend to think things like:

If I blush, people will think . . .

❑ I'm anxious and weak

❑ I fancy them

❑ I'm not telling the truth

❑ I'm hiding something

❑ I'm weird

❑ I'm childish

What does blushing mean to most people?

Over the years, we have done many surveys of hundreds of young people and adults about what they really think about blushing. Interestingly, the ideas above just don't come up. What most people tend to say is that they don't pay much attention to blushing. Blushing is not headline news to them. Most say that if they do notice somebody blushing they might think they are hot, maybe a little embarrassed. People say they find it endearing. They don't tend to think in the same negative way about it as those of us who fear blushing do. People don't think of blushing as weird or as a sign of weakness.

What might keep us trapped worrying about a blush?

When we worry about blushing we tend to focus more on ourselves than we do on the task at hand. This can make us feel even more self-conscious. Once again, our sneaky behaviour traps also keep us stuck fearing blushing. Take a look at the table below which shows some common behaviour traps people use when they fear blushing. Which might you use? What might the impact of these traps be?

For example, Nita realised that she tended to put her head down and use her hair to cover her face if she felt she was blushing. This meant that she never saw how others responded. If anything, it brought more attention to her.

Common behaviour traps when we feel we are blushing	Ways they may be keeping me trapped
	Without our awareness, these can:
• Cover face/neck/chest	• Make me feel more self-conscious
• Wear hair down	• Mean that I never see how others respond
• Look away/bend down	• Possibly draw more attention to me
• Wear make-up	• Stop others from getting to know me
• Divert attention away from myself	
• Keep quiet	
• Focus on myself, not others	
Others:	Others:

Do others notice a blush?

When we feel we are blushing, it can feel like we stand out from the crowd. Like we are suddenly wearing a red nose on our face and everybody can see. We might have a picture in our mind of how we think it looks. For example, seeing yourself with bright red or shiny cheeks. However, is blushing as noticeable as it feels?

We know from studies we have done filming people with social anxiety that they tend to overestimate how noticeable a blush looks.

Because blushing is a fear of yours, you are more focused on it than others are. You probably see it in your mind as looking more noticeable than it does. To others it may not be visible. Even if it is noticeable, it is not headline news to most people.

What would you say to a friend?

If you had a friend who occasionally blushed, would you think they were weird or weak? Would it make you decide you didn't want to know them? If somebody really rejected somebody else because of a blush – would that be the kind of person you would respect and want to be mates with? Try to keep in mind that in your worst-case scenario – somebody rejects you because of a blush – this is most likely not somebody worth knowing.

Take action

Confidence tasks to overcome a fear of blushing

1. Seeing blushing as a golden opportunity

 Any time from now on that you think you feel yourself blushing, grab that moment as a golden opportunity! Rather than looking down, hiding your face, keeping quiet, instead switch your focus to those around you. Observe them. How are they responding? Do they seem to have noticed? Are they responding negatively? Or do they carry on as usual? The more you can try this courageous step, the more data you will gather to overcome your fear of blushing. See Nita's log below:

👣 Step 1. Belief	👣 Step 2. Situation	👣 Step 3. Predict	👣 Step 4. Do it!	👣 Step 5. Reflect	👣 Step 6. Look ahead
Blushing – others will laugh.	Any time I feel I'm blushing this week.	If I blush, others will laugh and mention it – 70%.	Every time I feel like I'm blushing, don't hide – look up and observe how others react.	Monday: Felt like I was blushing in class, looked up, nobody laughed. Tuesday: Felt like I was blushing at lunch, kept talking, nobody seemed to notice. Wednesday: Felt like I was blushing talking to Dan; he didn't say anything about it. Re-rated prediction: Blushing means others will laugh – 20%.	I'll keep trying this. I'm realising that my blushing doesn't seem as noticeable to others. People seem to like me even when I feel I'm blushing.

Now it's your turn:

Step 1. Belief	Step 2. Situation	Step 3. Predict	Step 4. Do it!	Step 5. Reflect	Step 6. Look ahead	
What fearful belief will you focus on?	*What situation will you test out your fear in?*	*What is the worst that you think might happen?* *How would you know?* *0–100%*	*How will you test it out?* *Remember to get externally focused and drop behaviour traps.*	*What happened?* *Re-rate your prediction (0–100%).* *What does this tell you about yourself more generally?*	*What are you going to try next to build on your learning?*	

2. Standing up to the fear of blushing

A great confidence task is also to try doing something that you usually avoid because of your fear of blushing. Just remember to follow the two golden rules: drop those behaviour traps and get out of your head. For example, speaking up in class or making yourself a little more the centre of attention by dropping something on purpose in a busy area. This can be a great way to build your confidence: to show yourself that even if you feel self-conscious and as though you are blushing, it is most likely not as important to others as you feel it is.

Step 1. Belief	Step 2. Situation	Step 3. Predict	Step 4. Do it!	Step 5. Reflect	Step 6. Look ahead
Blushing – others will laugh.	When in the lunch line, drop my keys.	If I blush, others will laugh and mention it – 60%.	Rather than looking down and covering my face, look up and around as I pick the keys up. See how others respond.	A couple of people looked over, then carried on with their lunch. I felt hot in the face but nobody laughed or pointed it out. Re-rated prediction: Blushing means others will laugh – 20%.	Maybe my blushing is not as much of a big deal as I think. People don't care as much as I do. Carry on doing things I usually avoid and keep observing how others respond.

Now it's your turn:

Step 1. Belief	Step 2. Situation	Step 3. Predict	Step 4. Do it!	Step 5. Reflect	Step 6. Look ahead
What fearful belief will you focus on?	*What situation will you test out your fear in?*	*What is the worst that you think might happen?* *How would you know?* *0–100%*	*How will you test it out?* *Remember to get externally focused and drop behaviour traps.*	*What happened?* *Re-rate your prediction (0–100%).* *What does this tell you about yourself more generally?*	*What are you going to try next to build on your learning?*

3. What do others think about blushing?

Nita was keen to find out what her close friends might think about blushing. She decided to try something brave and say to a close friend, 'I really blushed when Miss Kelly asked me to speak up in class earlier,' to see what her friend would say. She was surprised to hear her friend say, 'Oh, I didn't notice. Yeah, I often blush when I'm put on the spot – I hate it when Miss Kelly picks on us like that.' You might want to try this yourself with a trusted friend or family member.

Make some notes about what you learnt below:

4. Is blushing as noticeable as it feels?

When working through Chapter 4, Seeing Myself in a More Positive Way, you might have already tried taking a video of yourself to see what you really look like when you feel you are blushing. If not, let's give this a try now.

You may already have some video of yourself when you felt you were blushing that you have avoided looking at until now. If not, you may want to ask somebody you trust to record some video. Or you could try pretending you are giving a talk in class about a recent holiday you went on and stand up and record yourself speaking for sixty seconds on your phone or laptop.

Remember the two golden rules of confidence tasks:

Golden rule 1: Drop your behaviour traps (so keep your head up and don't hide your face).

Golden rule 2: Get out of your head (so focus on the task at hand, not your feelings).

Before you watch the video back, make a prediction based on your feelings about how you think you will look. You might want to try finding something in the room that matches the shade you felt you looked (or google red colour charts). Then try watching the video back. Again, try to imagine you are watching a loved one speaking; try to ignore any self-critical thoughts and think of it as somebody else. Ask yourself:

- Does that person look like they are really anxious?

- If I was an alien coming down from space would I think that person looked bright red/shiny/(add in your prediction based on your feelings)?

- How does the video compare to my predictions based on my feelings?

- Try to ignore any self-critical thoughts – what would you say if it was your friend in the video? What would be your overall sense of how they looked?

- Is it possible you look like an acceptable person, much like everybody else?

Make some notes about what you learnt below:

Key points and giving yourself credit

Well done for working through this section on blushing. Take a moment to give yourself credit for working on this fear and for any of the confidence tasks you tried. A great way to build on your learning and to start being kinder to yourself is to make some notes on what you can give yourself credit for and what you learnt from it.

Nita's example:

What I can give myself credit for	Key learning points: Blushing
Reading through the section on blushing.	• Blushing is a part of being human. • It is the meaning I give to it that makes it a problem for me. • Focusing on myself and my behaviour traps are keeping me trapped fearing blushing.
Trying my confidence tasks: Using the feeling of a blush as a golden opportunity to drop my behaviour traps and focus on how others react.	• If I drop my behaviour traps when I feel I'm blushing, others don't respond as negatively as I think.
Standing up to the fear of blushing by doing something I usually avoid, dropping my behaviour traps and observing how others respond. Finding out what others think of blushing by dropping it into the conversation. Finding out if I blush as much as I feel by watching myself on video.	• Others don't seem to notice blushing as I much as I think they will. • Blushing is not headline news to others. • I don't blush as much as I think I do. • I look totally acceptable when I feel I'm blushing.

Now it's your turn:

What I can give myself credit for	Key learning points: Blushing

Feeling shaky

'I'm shaking'

'Others will see me shake'

It might surprise you to know that every person has a natural shake in their muscles. It is part of being human! If you ask anybody to hold their hand out and balance a piece of paper on top of it you will see the paper wobbling a little. If you don't believe us, give this a try! You could also ask a family member or close friend who doesn't worry about shaking to try it. You will discover that we all shake a little. We can also all feel more shaky at different times. Here are a few common reasons:

- Carrying something heavy

- Holding something tightly for a long time

- If our muscles are overworked

- Got a fever

- Low blood sugar levels

- Drinking drinks with too much caffeine

- Feeling stressed or had a shock

- Focusing too much on how shaky we feel (the more we focus on something the more we notice it)

But if we all feel shaky at times, why do some of us worry about shaking more than others?

What does feeling shaky mean to you?

Those people who worry less about feeling shaky tend to brush it off as something that happens to everybody at times. They may not even notice it happening. Those of us who fear shaking tend to think things like:

If I shake, people will see it and think. . .

❑ I'm anxious and weak

❑ I'm weird

❑ There's something wrong with me

We may worry that others will point it out and laugh.

What does shaking mean to most people?

Over the years, we have done many surveys of hundreds of young people and adults about what they really think about shaking. Interestingly, what we find is that people don't pay much attention to shaking. It is not such a big deal to them. Most say that if they do notice somebody shaking they might think they are feeling unwell and they don't dwell on it. They don't tend to think in the same negative way about it as those of us who fear shaking do.

What might keep us trapped worrying about shaking?

Those of us who worry about shaking tend to focus on how shaky or not we feel, rather than getting lost in the social situation. We also can fall into those tricky behaviour traps. Take a look at the table below which shows some common traps people use when they fear shaking. Which might you use? What might the impact of these traps be?

For example, Nita tended to grip things tightly when she felt her hands shaking. She would also look down. She realised that holding things so tightly might make her feel more shaky, and by looking down she never found out if others even noticed it.

Common behaviour traps when we feel we are shaky	Ways they may be keeping me trapped
	Without our awareness, these can:
• Look down	• Make me feel more shaky
• Grip things tightly	• Mean that I never see how others respond
• Hide my hands	• Possibly draw more attention to me
• Divert attention away from myself	• Stop others from getting to know me
• Keep quiet	
• Monitor how shaky or not my hands feel	
• Check if I am shaking or not	
• Focus on myself, not others	
Others:	Others:

What would you say to a friend?

Picture this – you are talking to a friend and you notice their hand shake slightly. Would you decide they were weird and you shouldn't speak to them again? If somebody really rejected somebody else because they shook a bit, would that be somebody you would want in your life? Do they sound like good friendship material? Try to keep in mind that in your worst-case scenario – somebody rejects you because you shake – this is most likely not somebody you would want to hang out with.

Take action

Confidence tasks to overcome a fear of shaking

1. What might be trapping me feeling shaky?
Find out for yourself

 One of the most common traps we use when feeling shaky is to grip things more tightly. This backfires because it can make us feel shakier.

To find this out for yourself, start by holding a cup loosely and asking yourself how shaky you feel from 0–100%. Then grip the cup tightly for a few minutes. Then rate how shaky you feel again from 0–100%. Compare your experiences. What most people discover is that when gripping things tightly they feel shakier! The shakiness is often driven by the behaviour trap itself.

Another common behaviour trap people use is to monitor (keep checking) how shaky their hands feel. This can also backfire by making us feel our hands are more weak or shaky.

A quick way to show yourself this is to hold your hands up in front of you. Spend a few minutes asking yourself, *How do my hands feel?* Focus all your attention on your hands. What you will notice is that, after a short while, your hands might start to feel unusual, strange, weaker or shaky. Simply by focusing too much on our hands we can feel shakier. Once again – it is our behaviour traps that can make us feel shakier.

Make some notes about what you learnt below:

2. *Feeling shaky is a golden opportunity*

Any time from now on that you think you feel yourself shaking, grab that moment as a golden opportunity! Rather than looking down, hiding your hands, keeping quiet, gripping things tightly, instead switch your focus to those around you. Observe others. How are they responding? Do they seem to have noticed anything unusual? Are they responding negatively? Or do they carry on as usual? The more you can try this courageous step – the more data you will gather to overcome your fear of shaking. See Nita's log below:

👣 Step 1. Belief	👣 Step 2. Situation	👣 Step 3. Predict	👣 Step 4. Do it!	👣 Step 5. Reflect	👣 Step 6. Look ahead
I'm shaking – others will see and will laugh.	Any time I feel I'm shaking this week.	If I shake, others will notice and laugh or tease me – 70%.	Every time I feel like I'm shaking, don't hide hands – look up and observe how others react. Don't grip things tightly.	Monday: Felt like I was shaking when I was talking to friends. Carried on talking. Nobody said anything. Tuesday: Felt shaky speaking in a tutorial, spoke anyway, nobody laughed. Wednesday: Felt shaky drinking	I seem to be finding that others don't pay attention to me when I feel I'm shaking. It might not be as noticeable as I think – If I keep going with this I think my confidence will grow more.

at lunch, carried on holding cup loosely, nobody seemed to notice. I'm shaking – others will see and will laugh – 25%.	

Now it's your turn:

Step 1. Belief	Step 2. Situation	Step 3. Predict	Step 4. Do it!	Step 5. Reflect	Step 6. Look ahead
What fearful belief will you focus on?	*What situation will you test out your fear in?*	*What is the worst that you think might happen?* *How would you know?* 0–100%	*How will you test it out?* *Remember to get externally focused and drop behaviour traps.*	*What happened?* *Re-rate your prediction (0–100%).* *What does this tell you about yourself more generally?*	*What are you going to try next to build on your learning?*

3. Standing up to the fear of shaking

You have probably avoided doing lots of things because of your fear of shaking. One way to stand up to your fear is to try doing some of these things, without your behaviour traps. For example, drinking a drink in front of a group of others or speaking up in class while holding something. This can be a great way to build your confidence, to show yourself that even if you feel shaky it is most likely not as noticeable to others.

👣 Step 1. Belief	👣 Step 2. Situation	👣 Step 3. Predict	👣 Step 4. Do it!	👣 Step 5. Reflect	👣 Step 6. Look ahead
Shaking – others will see and think I'm odd.	Drink a can of Coke in front of my friends.	If I shake, they will give me an odd look and walk away – 60%.	Drink a can of Coke when talking to others at break. Hold can loosely. Focus on them, not myself.	I felt shaky but nobody stared or gave me an odd look. They all spoke to me all break. Shaking – others will see and think I'm odd – 30%.	Maybe they didn't notice it. I'm accepted even if I feel shaky. Keep trying this out this week whenever I can.

Now it's your turn:

Step 1. Belief	Step 2. Situation	Step 3. Predict	Step 4. Do it!	Step 5. Reflect	Step 6. Look ahead
What fearful belief will you focus on?	*What situation will you test out your fear in?*	*What is the worst that you think might happen?*	*How will you test it out?*	*What happened?*	*What are you going to try next to build on your learning?*
		How would you know?	*Remember to get externally focused and drop behaviour traps.*	*Re-rate your prediction (0–100%).*	
		0–100%		*What does this tell you about yourself more generally?*	

4. *What do others think about shaking?*

Nita was keen to find out what people might think about shaking. When she was in the line for the bus, she pretended to speak to somebody on the phone saying, 'I was so shaky when I gave my presentation in class earlier', loud enough for those around to hear. As she said it, she looked around, expecting others to give her a weird look and laugh, but nobody paid her much attention. It didn't seem to be head-line news to them. You might want to try this yourself or try sharing this with a trusted friend or family member to see how they respond.

Make some notes about what you learnt below:

5. *Is shaking as noticeable as it feels?*

You might have already tried taking a video of yourself to see what you really look like when you feel you are shaking, as we covered this in Chapter 4. If not, let's give this a try now.

You may already have a video of yourself from a time you felt shaky. If not, you may want to ask somebody you trust to take some video. Or you could try pretending you are presenting to your class and record yourself talking for a minute or two on your phone or laptop. If you usually avoid holding things for fear of shaking, then hold something (like a cup or pen) loosely, without trying to avoid shaking.

Golden rule 1: Drop our behaviour traps (so don't grip anything tightly or hide the parts of you that you worry will shake).

Golden rule 2: Get out of your head (so focus on the task at hand, not your feelings).

Before you watch the video back, make a prediction based on your feelings about how you think you will look (e.g., my hands will shake 70%). Then try watching the video back. Again, try to imagine you are watching a loved one speaking, try to ignore any self-critical thoughts and think of it as somebody else. Ask yourself:

- Does that person look like they are really anxious?

- If I was an alien coming down from space would I think that person looked 70% shaky (add in your prediction based on your feelings)?

- How does the video compare to my predictions based on my feelings?

- Try to ignore any self-critical thoughts – what would you say if it was your friend in the video? What would your overall sense of how they looked be?

- Is it possible you look like an acceptable person, much like everybody else?

Make some notes about what you learnt below:

Key points and giving yourself credit

 Well done for working through this section on feeling shaky. Take a moment to give yourself credit for working on this fear and for any of the confidence tasks you tried. A great way to build on your learning and to start being kinder to yourself is to make some notes on what you can give yourself credit for and what you learnt from it.

Nita's example:

What I can give myself credit for	Key learning points: Shaking
Reading through the section on feeling shaky.	• Everybody's muscles shake a little. • It is the meaning I give to it that makes it a problem for me. • Focusing on myself and my behaviour traps are keeping me trapped fearing shaking.
Trying my confidence tasks: Using feeling shaky as a golden opportunity to drop my behaviour traps and observe how others react. Standing up to the fear of shaking by doing something I tend to avoid and dropping behaviour traps. Find out what others think of shaking by dropping it into the conversation. Find out if I look as shaky as I feel by watching myself on video.	• If I drop my behaviour traps when I feel I'm shaking, others don't respond as negatively as I think. • Others don't seem to notice it when I feel shaky. • Shaking is not headline news to others. • When I feel shaky, it doesn't look as shaky as it feels. • I look like a normal person even when I feel shaky inside. My feelings aren't visible.

Now it's your turn:

What I can give myself credit for	Key learning points: Shaking

Fear of sweating

'I'm sweating'

'Others will see me sweat'

If you are alive – you sweat. It is our body's way of cooling down. If you do a Google Image search for 'sweaty celebrities', you will see well-known faces of all backgrounds sweating. We simply cannot avoid it. Some of us may sweat more when:

- Hot

- Exercising

- We have fast metabolism

- Dehydrated

- Rushing

- Feeling nervous or stressed

- Going through hormonal changes

- Running a temperature/unwell

But if we all sweat at times, why do some of us worry about it more than others?

What does sweating mean to you?

Those people who worry less about feeling sweaty probably pay it little attention when it happens. Those of us who fear sweating tend to think things like:

If I sweat people will see it and think . . .

❏ I'm anxious and weak

❏ I'm weird

❏ There's something wrong with me

❏ I'm disgusting, I smell

We may worry others will point it out and laugh.

What does sweating mean to most people?

We have done many surveys of young people and adults about what they really think about sweating. We find that sweating is not such a big deal to the average person. Most say that if they do notice somebody sweating they might think they are hot, but they don't think much more about it than that.

What might keep us trapped worrying about sweating?

When we feel sweaty, we tend to focus more on how hot and sweaty we feel than we do on the people we are talking to. We can also fall back on behaviour traps that keep us stuck worrying about sweating. Take a look at the table below which shows some common traps people use when they fear sweating. Which might you use? What might the impact of these traps be?

For example, Josh realised he tended to cover sweat by wearing extra layers, which actually made him sweat more.

Common behaviour traps when we fear sweating	Ways they may be keeping me trapped
	Without our awareness, these can:
• Wear extra layers	• Make me feel hotter and sweat more
• Wear dark clothes	• Mean that I never see how others respond
• Keep arms down	• Possibly draw more attention to me
• Wipe sweat away	• Make me more aware of how sweaty I feel
• Try to keep cool	• Make it harder for me to cool down
• Monitor how sweaty I feel	• Stop others from getting to know me
• Avoid eye contact or talking to others if I feel sweaty	
• Focus on myself, not others	
Others:	Others:

What would you say to a friend?

Imagine you are at a party and you see a friend of yours is sweating. Would you decide they were disgusting and you shouldn't speak to them again? If somebody really rejected somebody else because they noticeably sweat, do they sound like good friendship material? If somebody rejects you because you sweat – this is most likely not somebody you would respect or be friends with.

Take action

Confidence tasks to overcome a fear of sweating

1. Feeling sweaty is a golden opportunity

 Every time from now on that you think you feel yourself sweating, grab that moment as a golden opportunity! Rather than looking down, trying to wipe away or cover your sweat, or hiding away, instead switch your focus to those around you. Observe others. How are they responding? Do they seem to have noticed anything unusual? Are they responding negatively? Or do they carry on as usual? The more you can try this courageous step, the more data you will gather to overcome your fear of sweating. See Josh's learning below:

Step 1. Belief	Step 2. Situation	Step 3. Predict	Step 4. Do it!	Step 5. Reflect	Step 6. Look ahead
I'm sweating – others will see and think I'm weird.	Any time I feel sweaty this week.	If I sweat, others will notice, think I'm disgusting and weird and give me a weird look, then leave – 60%.	Every time I feel like I'm sweating, don't hide, carry on the chat, don't cover my armpits or keep arms down. Observe how others react.	Monday: Felt sweaty at lunch but sat with friends anyway. Nobody seemed to notice. Tuesday: Felt sweaty in class. Spoke to the person sitting next to me anyway. Didn't leave or look disgusted. Wednesday: Felt sweaty talking to teacher. They didn't seem to notice or care. I'm sweating – others will see and think I'm weird – 30%.	Even though I felt sweaty a lot, nobody seemed to leave or look disgusted. It might not be as noticeable as I think. Keep going – confidence will grow too!

Now it's your turn:

Step 1. Belief	Step 2. Situation	Step 3. Predict	Step 4. Do it!	Step 5. Reflect	Step 6. Look ahead	
What fearful belief will you focus on?	*What situation will you test out your fear in?*	*What is the worst that you think might happen? How would you know? 0–100%*	*How will you test it out? Remember to get externally focused and drop behaviour traps.*	*What happened? Re-rate your prediction (0–100%). What does this tell you about yourself more generally?*	*What are you going to try next to build on your learning?*	

2. *Standing up to the fear of sweat*

Josh avoided lots of things because of his fear of sweating – like talking to people he liked, wearing light T-shirts or being the centre of attention. Like Josh, there might be lots of things you avoid doing because of your fear of sweating. The route to overcoming your fear is to do some of the things you tend to avoid, without your behaviour traps. For example, wear a light-coloured shirt when you meet up with friends, talk to somebody when you are feeling hot and sweaty. See what Josh did below:

Step 1. Belief	Step 2. Situation	Step 3. Predict	Step 4. Do it!	Step 5. Reflect	Step 6. Look ahead
Sweating – others will see and think I'm weird and disgusting.	Wear a light grey T-shirt around mates.	If I sweat, it will be noticeable and they will think I'm disgusting, give me an odd look and make an excuse to leave – 50%.	Keep talking even if I feel hot and sweaty. Focus on them, not myself. Don't hide.	I felt hot and sweaty and I think it was noticeable a bit but I kept chatting to my mates and nobody left or gave me a disgusted look – 20%.	It is probably more noticeable to me than others. They seem to like me even if I sweat. Try this again to build my confidence.

Now it's your turn:

Step 1. Belief	Step 2. Situation	Step 3. Predict	Step 4. Do it!	Step 5. Reflect	Step 6. Look ahead
What fearful belief will you focus on?	*What situation will you test out your fear in?*	*What is the worst that you think might happen?* *How would you know?* *0–100%*	*How will you test it out?* *Remember to get externally focused and drop behaviour traps.*	*What happened?* *Re-rate your prediction (0–100%).* *What does this tell you about yourself more generally?*	*What are you going to try next to build on your learning?*

3. What do others think about sweating?

Josh wanted to find out what others thought about sweating. When talking to a good friend, he threw into the chat that he got really sweaty talking to somebody he liked earlier that day. His friend smiled and said, 'I knew you liked them!' but didn't seem to care that he had got sweaty. You might want to try this yourself or try sharing this with a trusted friend or family member to see how they respond.

Make some notes about what you learnt below:

4. Is sweating as noticeable as it feels?

You might have already tried taking a video of yourself to see what you really look like when you feel you are sweaty, as we covered this in Chapter 4. If not, let's give this a try now.

You may already have a photo or video of yourself from a time you felt sweaty that you have avoided looking at. If not, you may want to ask somebody you trust to take some video. Or you could try pretending you are presenting to your class and record yourself talking for a minute or two on your phone or laptop. Remember the golden rules:

Golden rule 1. Drop our behaviour traps (so don't hide or wipe away any sweat; wear clothes that would show it).

Golden rule 2: Get out of our heads (so focus on the task at hand, not our feelings).

Before you watch the video back, make a prediction based on your feelings about how you think you will look (e.g. I will look 80% sweaty). Then try watching the video back. Again, try to imagine you are watching a loved one speaking, try to ignore any self-critical thoughts and think of it as somebody else. Ask yourself:

- Does that person look like they are really anxious?

- If I was an alien coming down from space would I think that person looked 80% sweaty (add in your prediction based on your feelings)?

- How does the video compare to my predictions based on my feelings?

- Try to ignore any self-critical thoughts – what would you say if it was your friend in the video? What would your overall sense of how they looked be?

- Is it possible you look like an acceptable person, much like everybody else?

Make some notes about what you learnt below:

Key points and giving yourself credit

 Well done for working through this section on feeling sweaty. Take a moment to give yourself credit for working on this fear and for any of the confidence tasks you tried. A great way to build on your learning and to start being kinder to yourself is to make some notes on what you can give yourself credit for and what you learnt from it.

For example:

What I can give myself credit for	Key learning points: Feeling sweaty
Reading through the section on feeling sweaty.	• Everybody sweats. It is part of being human. • It is the meaning I give to sweating that makes it a problem for me. • Focusing on myself and my behaviour traps are keeping me trapped fearing sweating.
Trying my confidence tasks: Using feeling sweaty as a golden opportunity to find out how others respond. Standing up to the fear of sweating by dropping my behaviour traps and observing others.	• If I drop my behaviour traps when I feel sweaty, others don't respond as negatively as I think. • Others don't seem to notice it when I feel sweaty.
Find out what others think of sweating by dropping it into conversation. Find out if it is as noticeable as it feels by watching myself on video.	• Sweating is not headline news to others. It's part of being human. • When I feel sweaty it doesn't look as noticeable as it feels. • I look like a normal person even when I feel sweaty. • My feelings aren't visible.

Now it's your turn:

What I can give myself credit for	Key learning points: Feeling Sweaty

Feeling like I'm unacceptable (weird – unlikeable – not good enough)

'I'm not good enough'

'I'm weird' 'I'm unlikeable' 'I'm different'

It can be really painful to feel that you are weird, different, unlikeable or not good enough, and maybe it's hard even to acknowledge that you have these thoughts. But if you do feel this way, you are far from alone. These are some of the most common thoughts young people with social anxiety have.

When you are in a social situation, rather than an enjoyable experience does it feel like you are in front of a panel of tough judges? As if you are being scrutinised and likely to come up short? Lots of young people tell us they feel this way. But is this how social situations really work? Take a moment to think about what goes through your mind when you spend time with others. Are you rating how likeable they are? Are you judging how weird they are? Thinking about whether they are good enough? Do you often walk away having come to this conclusion about others?

Most of us don't think about others in this way. We focus on what went on in the interaction – we might think, *That was a nice chat, We got on well* or, *We didn't have much to talk about.* We don't spend our time ranking people.

Young people often fear others will conclude they are weird or unlikeable if they show signs of anxiety or don't say much. Ask yourself: *What would you make of these signs or qualities if you noticed them in somebody else?* Like most people, you probably wouldn't conclude that the person was totally unlikeable or weird.

In fact, when we have done surveys asking people what would make them think of somebody as **unlikeable**, they respond with things like:

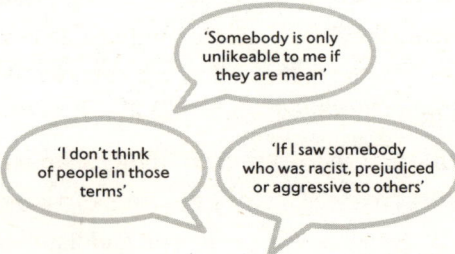

'Somebody is only unlikeable to me if they are mean'

'I don't think of people in those terms'

'If I saw somebody who was racist, prejudiced or aggressive to others'

And when we have done surveys asking people what would make them think of somebody as **weird**, they respond with things like:

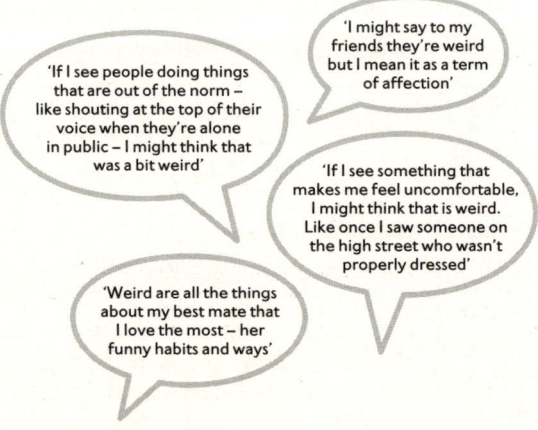

'I might say to my friends they're weird but I mean it as a term of affection'

'If I see people doing things that are out of the norm – like shouting at the top of their voice when they're alone in public – I might think that was a bit weird'

'If I see something that makes me feel uncomfortable, I might think that is weird. Like once I saw someone on the high street who wasn't properly dressed'

'Weird are all the things about my best mate that I love the most – her funny habits and ways'

You may often think of yourself as unlikeable or weird, but these are most likely thoughts and feelings you have about yourself, rather than what others are thinking.

It may be that others have put you down, or called you weird or unlikeable. If this is the case for you, it is understandable that you will have these fears. You might find Chapter 11, Dealing with Bullies or Teasing (in the Past or Present), helpful. Ask yourself, if somebody is going around telling another person they are weird or unlikeable – what does that say about them? Is that somebody you would respect? Would you think highly of them? If the answer is no, maybe they aren't the best judge. So, we should take a fresh look at these thoughts.

'I'm unlikeable or weird': Reviewing the week with fresh eyes

Hopefully you will have already learnt from this book that your own thoughts and feelings are not the most reliable evidence of what others are thinking. We would like you to consider the last week with fresh eyes. Rather than using your feelings to judge, are there any signs, however small, that others might not think you are unlikeable or weird? Is there any evidence you are acceptable or OK as you are?

You may have tried other confidence tasks recommended in this book and discovered evidence that others accept you more than you thought. You might want to add some of that evidence below too. For example, if you tried the staring experiment (in the section on feeling stared at in this chapter or earlier in Chapter 3), did you discover that people stare at you as if you are weird/different/stand out? Or in fact, did you find that people treat you just like anybody else walking down the street?

If you find this tricky, consider what you would say if you were talking to a good friend who felt this way about themselves.

Nita wrote things down like: *I got invited along to the cinema. When I spoke to Kate at the gym she responded well. I talked a bit more when speaking to friends in class the other day and they didn't give me a weird look or ignore me.*

Any evidence over the week I am more acceptable than I feel I am

If you find yourself thinking of a time you did feel unlikeable, weird or unacceptable, try asking yourself whether there could be another way of looking at that moment now with fresh eyes? Focus only on the evidence (ignore that inner critic or those feelings!).

Nita added: *When I went to a party the other week, I left early as I felt anxious and I assumed everybody thought I was unlikeable and it was weird I left. Looking at it with fresh eyes, I didn't really give people a chance. People were probably too busy with the party to think much about the fact I left.*

If you struggled with the above, be kind to yourself. It is hard to start to think about things differently. If you have a good friend or family member you trust you might want to ask them to help you.

What keeps us stuck feeling this way about ourselves? Our self-focused attention and behaviour traps.

For many of us our behaviour traps and self-focused attention drive this way of seeing ourselves and keep us stuck.

Consider some common behaviour traps that can fuel **feeling unlikeable or weird/different:**

Common behaviour traps when we fear others think we are unlikeable

- Try to come across as 'likeable' by only saying things I think others will approve of

- Don't share much about myself

- Keep quiet in groups

- Try to please others – avoid saying no or disagreeing with others

Others:

Ways they may be keeping me trapped

Without our awareness, these can:

- Make it hard for me to feel acceptable/liked for who I am

- Make it hard for others to get to know me

- Mean that I don't build deeper connections with people

- Make me feel inferior

Others:

Consider some common behaviour traps that can fuel **feeling weird/odd or different:**

Common behaviour traps when we fear others think we are weird, different or odd	Ways they may be keeping me trapped
	Without our awareness, these can:
• Try to act normal and not stand out	• Mean I'm not really my full self with others – so I don't feel accepted
• Try to blend in (e.g. wear dark clothes)	• Make it hard for others to get to know me
• Watch everything I say and only say things I think sound 'normal'	• Mean that I don't build deeper connections with people
• Keep quiet in groups	• Mean I always feel different
• Monitor how weird/different I am all the time	• Make me feel inferior
• Compare myself unfairly to others	
Others:	Others:

Discovering the impact of self-focused attention and behaviour traps. One way to discover the impact of self-focused attention and behaviour traps on how unlikeable or weird we feel is to spend a few minutes talking to a friend or family member using a couple of your behaviour traps (such as keeping quiet), focusing on yourself and repeatedly asking yourself, 'How unlikeable am I?' or, 'How weird am I coming across?' What you will find is that this can quickly increase how unlikeable or weird you feel. Instead, when you get out of your head and get lost in the conversation, these feelings should start to reduce.

Feeling unlikeable or weird is not a reflection of what others are thinking. It is often a product of your self-focus and behaviour traps.

Take action

Confidence tasks to overcome feeling unlikeable or weird

1. Share a little more of yourself to break free from your fears

 As we discovered above, our behaviour traps and self-focused attention can keep us stuck fearing that others think of us as unlikeable and weird. The best way to break free from these fears is to drop our behaviour traps and share a little more of ourselves. So, if you usually don't say much and keep quiet, share a little more in a conversation. If you prepare or watch what you do say to try to come across as likeable or normal, try saying whatever comes to mind.

See what Josh did:

Step 1. Belief	Step 2. Situation	Step 3. Predict	Step 4. Do it!	Step 5. Reflect	Step 6. Look ahead
I'm unlikeable.	Chatting to friends at school during break.	If I share a bit more about myself when we talk – like my weekend plans – then I think they will think I'm boring and unlikeable – 80%. They will ignore me and probably walk away.	I will talk a bit more about myself and see how they respond. Focus on them, not myself.	I talked a bit about my weekend plans and they talked about theirs. I felt like I shared more about myself and that felt good. Nobody ignored me. I'm unlikeable and boring – 40%.	I will keep trying to talk a little more about myself so friends get to know me more.

Now it's your turn:

Step 1. Belief	Step 2. Situation	Step 3. Predict	Step 4. Do it!	Step 5. Reflect	Step 6. Look ahead	
What fearful belief will you focus on?	What situation will you test out your fear in?	What is the worst that you think might happen? How would you know? 0–100%	How will you test it out? Remember to get externally focused and drop behaviour traps.	What happened? Re-rate your prediction (0–100%). What does this tell you about yourself more generally?	What are you going to try next to build on your learning?	

2. Using your feelings as a golden opportunity

Every time from now on that you think you feel weird, different or unlikeable, use that feeling as a golden opportunity! Rather than looking down, trying to act normal, or keeping quiet, instead switch your focus to those around you and get a little more involved in the chat/situation than you were. Observe others. How are they responding? Do they seem to have noticed anything unusual? Are they responding negatively? Or do they carry on as usual? The more you can try this courageous step, the more data you will gather to overcome your fears. See Josh's learning below:

Step 1. Belief	Step 2. Situation	Step 3. Predict	Step 4. Do it!	Step 5. Reflect	Step 6. Look ahead
I'm weird and unlikeable.	Any time I feel weird or unlikeable.	If I keep talking to others when I feel like I'm weird or unlikeable, they will give me a strange look or move away from me – 50%.	Every time I feel weird, like I don't fit in or am unlikeable, don't hide. Instead, carry on the chat. Observe how others react.	Monday: Felt unlikeable when talking to a friend in class but I carried on chatting. They didn't respond negatively. Tuesday: Felt weird when in a group but rather than looking down I kept my head up and nobody was giving me a weird look. Wednesday: Felt nobody liked me when playing football but I tried to ignore the feeling and chat to the others anyway. They chatted a bit and didn't ignore me. I'm weird and unlikeable – 20%.	Often when I get these feelings, if I ignore them and get lost in the situation I see that others don't respond in the negative way I feel they will. Just because I feel weird or unlikeable doesn't mean that's what others are thinking.

Now it's your turn:

Step 1. Belief	Step 2. Situation	Step 3. Predict	Step 4. Do it!	Step 5. Reflect	Step 6. Look ahead
What fearful belief will you focus on?	*What situation will you test out your fear in?*	*What is the worst that you think might happen?* *How would you know?* *0–100%*	*How will you test it out?* *Remember to get externally focused and drop behaviour traps.*	*What happened?* *Re-rate your prediction (0–100%).* *What does this tell you about yourself more generally?*	*What are you going to try next to build on your learning?*

Stop comparing yourself to others – you are good enough as you are

We hope that as you move through the chapters and try the confidence experiments in this book, you will start to feel more acceptable and good enough in social situations. In addition to the behaviour traps above, the feeling we are not good enough is fuelled by unfairly comparing ourselves to others and criticising ourselves. For example, Nita used to look at her friends when at a party and think, *I wish I found things as easy as them, I'm rubbish in comparison.* If this sounds familiar, it might be useful to keep in mind that most of us struggle with feeling not good enough at times. If you surveyed a room of people, it is unlikely that you would find anyone who would rate themselves as 100% confident, and our confidence can rise and fall at different times. Even people who appear outwardly confident don't always feel that way on the inside. The route to feeling good enough is to stop comparing yourself to others and be kinder to yourself. Keeping logs, like those above, and reading over them now and again can help. You will also find Chapter 8, Be Kind to Myself, helpful.

Key points and giving yourself credit

Well done for working through this section on feeling weird or unlikeable. Take a moment to give yourself credit for working on this fear and for any of the confidence tasks you tried.

A great way to build on your learning and to start being kinder to yourself is to make some notes on what you can give yourself credit for and what you learnt from it.

For example:

What I can give myself credit for	Key learning points: Feeling unlikeable or weird
Reading through the section on feeling weird or unlikeable.	• I may feel or think of myself as weird or unlikeable but this doesn't mean that is what others think of me. • Focusing on myself and my behaviour traps are keeping me trapped feeling different or unlikeable.
Trying my confidence tasks: Trying to look up and around if I notice myself feeling like I stand out and I'm being stared at. Sharing more of myself. Using feeling weird/ unlikeable as a golden opportunity to find out how others respond.	• The feeling of being weird and stared at comes from staring at myself. When I look up I see others aren't staring at me – I don't stand out in the negative way I feel I do. • If I drop my behaviour traps when I feel weird or unlikeable, others don't respond as negatively as I think.

Now it's your turn:

What I can give myself credit for	Key learning points: Feeling unlikeable or weird

Chapter 7

Confidence Experiments – The Next Step

Give your confidence a boost

'I'm still worried about what
others really think.'

'But what if I said something
really stupid?'

'What if I got really anxious
in front of the class?'

'Maybe it's not that noticeable . . .
but what if one day I get
really sweaty?'

Your confidence tasks have hopefully helped put some of your fears to the test. But you might still have some of the concerns above. When it comes to putting any fear behind us, the biggest confidence boost we can get is by facing our fears head-on.

In this chapter we are going to learn:

- How to take your confidence experiments further and face your fears head-on

- Suggestions for helpful experiments

If you feared the dark, you might need to spend some time in the dark to discover you could cope. If you feared heights, you would need to climb up to the top of a building.

When it comes to social fears, the route to freeing ourselves from our fears is to intentionally do some of the things that we fear might lead to our rejection or embarrassment and find out how others actually respond. It is by seeing that it is not a disaster, that others do not reject us, that we cope better than we think, and that we truly put our fears behind us and move forward. This probably sounds terrifying, so thanks for continuing to read on! You will be glad you did. Because we know from working with many hundreds of young people over the years how powerful these confidence-boosting tasks can be.

We recommend trying these tasks after you have given a few of the earlier confidence tasks a go.

Here are some examples of things Josh and Nita tried.

Josh's feeling 'boring' confidence boost: Josh was feeling more confident in himself after he had started to drop his behaviour traps and speak more spontaneously around his friends and in class. But he still had some worries. He thought if he really spoke at length about something less interesting, others would think he was dull and not want to hang out with him. He took a big leap forward by trying on purpose to talk about something he thought was dull. He spoke to his friend Mike for a long time about the fact his shower had broken at home. He tried to focus on Mike and observe how he reacted.

He predicted that Mike would think he was dull and make a quick escape. But he was surprised to discover that Mike joined in the chat, talking about how, at times, he couldn't shower for a weekend when he went camping and how much he hated it. The chat then moved on. But Mike didn't seem to care. Josh realised that even if his chat isn't that interesting, he was still accepted by his friends.

Nita's 'blushing' confidence boost: Nita was worrying less about blushing after some helpful confidence tasks. She was now keeping her hair back when she spoke and not looking down even if she felt she blushed. But she still worried that if she blushed when there were lots of people around she would be laughed at. She took a big leap forward when she decided to put a lot of blusher on her face to create the look of a blush and then go for a walk in her local shopping centre. She tried to keep her head up and focused on others, not herself.

She predicted that others would stare and point and laugh at her. She was shocked to see that nobody really noticed her. A couple of people glanced and then looked away. Nobody laughed at her. This was a huge boost to her confidence.

The table below gives a range of different social fears young people have and some suggestions of experiments you can try to overcome your fear and boost your confidence.

With each of these confidence-boosting tasks, remember to make a note of what your prediction is before you try the experiment. Make sure this is something you would see and observe, e.g. *I will see people laugh at me and say something negative*. The golden rules are slightly different here:

New golden rule 1: Purposefully do something that you fear would lead you to feel embarrassed or being rejected (ideas are in the table below). Try not to use your safety behaviours when you do this.

Golden rule 2: Get out of your head so you can check out how people respond to you.

You might be tempted to look down/away when you try something that makes you feel self-conscious, but it is at this moment that **it is key that you keep your head up and observe others around you!**

Confidence-boosting tasks – ideas list!

In the table below you will find a list of common fears and ideas of confidence-boosting tasks you could try. You could try these with friends, family or teachers. A number of them can be tried with people in public, shop assistants, etc. If you can, try these more than once to really give your confidence a boost.

Always focus on the other person, not yourself! Ignore how you feel and gather the evidence.

If you fear . . .	Confidence-boosting task	Example of what Nita/Josh tried
Being boring	Purposefully talk about something you think is boring.	Josh spoke to his mates at length about something he thought was boring – his shower not working.
Being stupid	Get something wrong on purpose/say something you think is stupid. Ask a shop assistant for something when it is in sight, e.g., 'Where is the ice cream?'	Nita told her friend she didn't know what gluten-free was (even though she did). Nita asked where the make-up was when she was right by it in a shop.
Freezing mid-conversation	Halfway through saying something, say, 'My mind has gone blank.'	Halfway through ordering a drink, Nita told the waitress her mind had gone blank, before carrying on her order.
Getting my words mixed up	Get your words mixed up on purpose.	Josh asked, 'Where are the games videos?' in a shop, before correcting himself: 'I meant video games.'

Pausing mid-conversation	Pause for a few seconds mid-sentence.	When asking her teacher a question, Nita paused for three seconds mid-sentence before carrying on.
Blushing	Put on some blusher or add Vaseline to create the look of a blush.	Nita put blusher on her cheeks and walked around her local shopping centre.
Shaking	Shake on purpose when around other people.	Nita shook her hands on purpose when drinking a Coke with friends at lunch.
Sweating	Add some water to your underarms or face to create the look of sweat.	Josh put water on his underarms so it was noticeable. He asked another student for directions to the art block, pointing to confirm the directions so his underarms could be seen.

Elyse's reflections

It helped me to start these confidence tasks with my close friends, and then I'd work my way out to people I felt less comfortable or familiar with. I think that really helped me build my confidence and discover that no one really cares.

I tried slipping up with my words or telling a wrong fact. That was a big one for me. I felt like I had to be correct all the time. I found out that no one's going to ridicule you for getting something slightly wrong in a conversation.

My confidence-boosting plan

Now it is your turn. In the record sheet below write down:

1. The beliefs/fears you want to test.
2. Situations you could test them in.
3. Your predictions (ignore feelings! What would you see/hear others do if your prediction was true?).
4. Then take a leap forward and try this out.
5. Reflect. Once you have done your tasks, make a note of what you learnt.
6. Note how you might want to take it a step forward by trying something else.

Remember, these are challenging tasks, but everybody we have worked with tells us that these are the tasks that really go on to set them free from their fears.

Step 1. Belief	Step 2. Situation	Step 3. Predict	Step 4. Do it!	Step 5. Reflect	Step 6. Look ahead
What fearful belief will you focus on?	What situation will you test out your fear in?	What is the worst that you think might happen? How would you know? 0–100%	How will you test it out? Remember to get externally focused and drop behaviour traps.	What happened? Re-rate your prediction (0–100%). What does this tell you about yourself more generally?	What are you going to try next to build on your learning?

Trying more challenging social tasks – public speaking

As your confidence starts to grow speaking to strangers and in groups you may want to take things a step further and work on building up your confidence when speaking to a larger audience (e.g. giving a talk in class).

If you feel anxious speaking up in front of an audience, you are far from alone. Public speaking is the most common human fear. You may look at other people and wonder why they seem to be able to do it so easily, but the chances are they also struggle with it. There are few people who feel totally at ease speaking up in front of people and those who do tend to have built up their confidence over time.

Everything we have covered in the book so far will help you build your confidence when speaking in front of other people. You may want to plan a confidence experiment to test out your fears when speaking in front of others. Our top tips for building your confidence giving presentations include:

- Focus on getting lost in the task, rather than on yourself.

- Spot any behaviour traps you use when speaking up in front of others or public speaking and experiment with dropping these.

- Remember, audiences work slightly differently to conversations. When giving a talk, the audience will rarely nod and smile. They can even look disinterested – but this is just how audiences work and not a reflection on you. Trust us: we give lectures regularly and know this first-hand! If you don't believe us, look around the class-room the next time a teacher presents. Importantly, when speaking to an audience, try not to be put off if people look less engaged – that's just what audiences look like.

Here are some common behaviour traps people find they fall into when public speaking, the possible impact of them and what you could try instead:

Common behaviour traps we use when speaking in front of an audience	Possible impact	What to try instead
Writing out a script in advance or rehearsing exactly what to say.	Makes it hard to get any words out.	Think of the key bullet points you want to cover and write these down on a Post-it note, and try speaking more spontaneously.
Avoiding eye contact.	Makes me more anxious.	Look at the audience as you speak.
Monitoring my speech.	Make me more self-conscious.	Say whatever comes to mind and focus on the task and the audience rather than what you have said.
Speaking quickly and avoiding pauses.	Puts huge pressure on myself.	Slow down a little and allow natural pauses.
Speaking quietly.	Makes it hard for people to follow what I'm saying.	Speak a little louder than you typically would and focus on the audience.

To build up your confidence public speaking you might want to try practising speaking about a topic of your choice (e.g. where you live, a holiday you enjoyed, a film you like, etc.) to a virtual audience while dropping your behaviour traps and self-focus. A virtual audience is a pre-recorded video of people listening to a talk or presentation. We have several different-sized virtual audiences online. Some are more challenging than others because they look less engaged with the speaker. You may want to start with the standard audience of three and build up to a larger, more challenging audience. You can find the links to the virtual audiences in the Resources section (page 360). We have found that doing this can start to build confidence in public speaking. Importantly, drop those behaviour traps and focus on the task at hand, rather than yourself!

Key points and giving yourself credit

 These confidence-boosting tasks are huge challenges – so be sure to give yourself a huge amount of credit for any you try. Imagine you are texting a good friend who had a fear and faced up to it in this way. Try reading that text back to yourself!

See what Nita wrote:

What I can give myself credit for	Key learning points
Wow, I was so brave. Even though I was terrified, I put blusher on my cheeks and walked through the shopping centre!	People didn't laugh or point it out like I feared. I showed myself that blushing is not major news – everybody is too caught up in themselves.
I shook my hand when drinking a Coke around some others at college. It was scary but I did it. I'm braver than I think I am! I'm going to give myself huge credit for this one.	They didn't pay much attention. I don't think people are as focused on my hands as I am. Maybe shaking isn't as big a deal as I feel it is and others don't think much about it.
I tried giving a talk to a virtual audience without overly planning what to say.	I found it easier to speak than when I usually script what to say! I'm going to try to experiment in my next class presentation with just bullet points of what to cover, but not writing it out sentence by sentence as I usually do.

Now it's your turn:

What I can give myself credit for	Key learning points

Chapter 8

Be Kind to Myself

Elyse's reflections

After I felt a social interaction went badly, I would get in a critical mindset and it would spiral fast. It would last for hours and hours and have a huge impact on me. Lots of people are hard on themselves as they think it motivates them. It helps to ask yourself: *Is this actually going to motivate me to change? Or is it just going to stop me from trying again?* To feel more confident I needed to speak to myself in a kinder, more constructive way.

In this chapter we are going to learn:

- About our inner voice and how friendly or critical ours is.

- How to break free from our inner critic.

- Tips on being kind to ourselves.

Do you have an inner friend or an inner critic?

Does Elyse's experience sound familiar to you? Imagine you make a joke with some friends and it just doesn't land. You might wish the floor would suddenly swallow you up – but what happens afterwards? Are you kind to your mind? Do you speak to yourself as you would to a good friend? Or do you beat yourself up – a bit like talking as your worst enemy?

Getting stuck going over and over moments we think we messed up is common. At these times we can speak to ourselves pretty harshly, kicking ourselves when we are already down. Most of us wouldn't dream of saying stuff we say to ourselves to anybody else because it would make them feel terrible!

Mistakes and mishaps are part of being human. There will always be times when things don't go to plan. But we can change the way we respond when this happens – we can learn to be kind to our mind, to lift our confidence rather than batter it down. In this chapter we will show you how.

Is your inner critic holding you back?

Research shows that many young people think putting themselves down is useful. You may find that you have some ideas of your own that being hard on yourself might stop a future mess-up or stop you getting big-headed. Let's take a moment to think about how helpful an inner critic really is . . .

Let's imagine you are about to start a new course and you are given a choice between two teachers:

Teacher A is super critical, puts students down and calls them names if they get things wrong. They never give encouragement if things go well. Achievements are ignored.

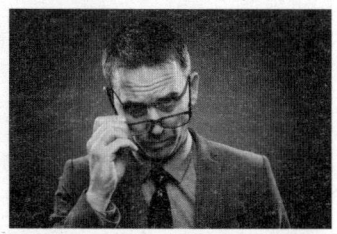

Teacher B is warm and encouraging. If mistakes are made, they support the student to learn a new way. They praise achievements.

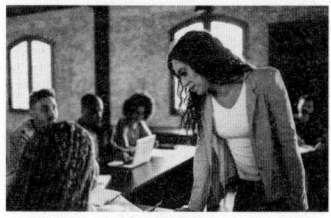

Which teacher would you prefer? We are guessing (hoping!) that you would prefer Teacher B. Why? Well, if any student had Teacher A they would surely be terrified. It would make them feel down and like it's impossible to learn.

Now think about how this applies to the way in which you speak to yourself when you think things go wrong. Self-criticism has the same impact on our emotions and our body as if we were verbally attacked by somebody else. Far from being useful, it can make us feel anxious and low and knocks our confidence. It can also make us assume that others are thinking in the same harsh and attacking way about us.

For example, after writing a post online, Josh found himself going over and over it. He started beating himself up: *You idiot. Why did you say that? Everybody must be thinking you are really weird.* Josh assumed his mates were also thinking he was an idiot. He felt low, anxious and like everybody was mocking him. Rather than speaking to his friends, Josh avoided them for the rest of the day. But most of his friends hadn't even seen his post, and those who had didn't think about it afterwards. He was stuck in a vicious cycle of being hard on himself and feeling worse and worse.

Do you ever get stuck in a similar cycle (like the one below)? If so, it is time to break free from it.

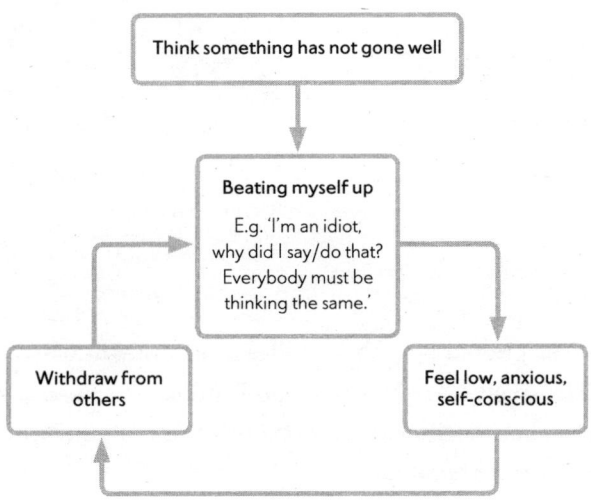

Time to break free from the inner critic

Spot the critic. Like a bully who follows you around, it may feel as though your inner critic is the boss – but it is time for you to take charge. The first step in breaking free from the critic is to notice when you are being hard on yourself and, rather than accepting it, call the critic out – name it.

Let's make a start on spotting your inner critic. Tick any of these common signs below that you notice when you are being hard on yourself:

❑ Calling myself names

❑ Speaking to myself harshly

❑ Telling myself off

❑ Questioning myself

❑ Feeling ashamed of myself

Name the critic. Now, when you notice these signs, ask yourself: *Is my inner critic speaking?* You may want to come up with your own name for it, e.g. my bully, my enemy, etc. Some people find it helpful to attach a picture to the name. Josh thought of his critic like a carousel ride he couldn't get off. He saved an image of a carousel as his phone screen-saver as a reminder to look out for the times he was stuck in a self-critical cycle.

Remind yourself of the downsides. It may be hard to let go of the inner critic if it is an old habit or if you have tended to see it as useful. It can be helpful to remind yourself of some of the downsides and why it will help to be kinder to yourself. Josh wrote himself a flashcard on his phone that he could look at when he spotted he was beating himself up.

Looking at this helped him to let go of the critic and start to speak to himself with more kindness.

My inner critic . . .

- Kicks me when I'm down

- Makes me feel low

- Stops me sleeping

- Steals my confidence

- Makes me see myself more negatively

If I can speak to myself with kindness, it might gradually build my confidence and help me feel better.

You might want to try adding a similar flashcard to your phone or in a notebook now.

Elyse's reflections

For me, I needed to spot the spiral of self-critical thoughts, take a step back and try to spot what I was thinking and re-evaluate. To ask myself: *Is this the way that I wanna be talking to myself? Is it going be beneficial for me? Is it going to make me feel better or worse by thinking this way a lot of the time?*

Being your own best friend (not your own worst enemy)

We are going to guess that you are probably better at being kind to others than you are to yourself. So here is a task to draw on those strengths that will help you learn to be kind to your own mind.

Imagine a close friend or loved one is saying the following to themselves. What would you tell them?

If you need a hand doing this, here is an example of one of the responses Nita wrote:

* Give yourself a break! People will be much less focused on it than you are. Go and do something nice for yourself to take your mind off it.

Your friend says . . .	Kinder response you would tell your friend
I didn't know the answer to a question in class today; everybody will be talking about how stupid I am.	
I didn't know the band people were talking about today; they will think I'm boring and uncool.	
I felt anxious giving a talk today; people will think I'm weird.	

Now, try reading these statements out to yourself the next time you catch your inner critic speaking to you. You might want to write a few of these down on your phone notes so you can access them wherever you are.

What are others really thinking?

For those times when you just cannot switch off from going over and over something that just happened in a critical way, it might help to take a step back and ask yourself what others might really be thinking.

In the moment it can feel like we are front and centre stage in somebody else's mind. However, this is often the inner critic deceiving you. The reality is usually the opposite.

A recent study analysing scans of people's brains has estimated that the average young person has around 6,000 thoughts a day! So even if people have had the odd negative thought about you, this is quickly lost in the sea of thousands of other thoughts. It is a drop in the ocean.

Take a moment to think about all the kinds of things other young people have on their minds. We find it helpful to draw the shape of a person's head on paper and write all the different things inside. Of course you will probably not guess all 6,000 thoughts! But hopefully it will give you an idea of how you are only one drop in the ocean of their mind. See our example below for ideas:

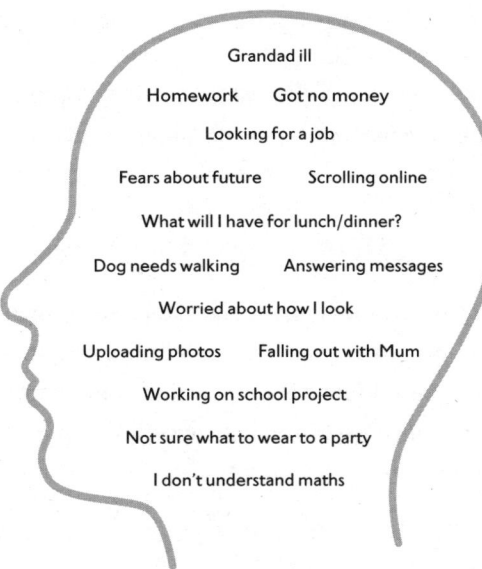

The next time you find yourself assuming everybody is criticising you as your inner critic does – take a look at this drawing. You might want to take a photo of it on your phone so you can find it any time you need it.

Elyse's reflections

Doing this task can help you see that although you might be thinking that something you said is front and centre in somebody else's head, it is a bit more like a grain of sand: much smaller to them than it felt to you.

Be kind, rewind

We have another helpful exercise here if you have tried the above and just cannot switch off from going over and over something. We sometimes call it 'Be kind, rewind'. You might recall doing a similar exercise earlier in this book in Chapter 4, Seeing Myself in a More Positive Way, page 66.

In this exercise, we will try going over the event you are being hard on yourself about in a different way. By rewinding it and being kind – focusing more on the facts, rather than on your feelings or critical thoughts. We are going to try to picture a recent social situation through the view of a camera, seeing only what is visible, not how you felt or thought about it.

Think about a recent time when you **felt** socially anxious and as if you came across in a negative way. Write out briefly what happened in the box below, and try to include:

- How you were feeling

- How you saw yourself in your own mind

- Any self-critical thoughts

- What happened next

- How others actually responded to you (i.e. what they did or said)

This is what Josh wrote:

> I was talking to a mate after going to the cinema and found myself feeling anxious that I didn't have much to say. I felt like I said something really dull to him. I was thinking I was such a boring idiot. I found myself feeling really anxious and self-conscious. I looked down and made an excuse to leave.

My example:

Now, let's imagine that a camera caught the whole thing on video. Read over what you wrote above and then cross out anything that would **not** be picked up by the camera.

- Cross out anything you felt inside your body that the camera wouldn't see, e.g. feeling sweaty, feeling red, feeling shaky, feeling anxious

- Cross out any self-critical thoughts you had about how you came across, e.g. 'I was boring', etc.

- Leave only factual evidence in the account, e.g. how others responded and what happened next

Here is Josh's account after he has crossed out anything that a camera would not see (his thoughts and feelings), leaving only the facts:

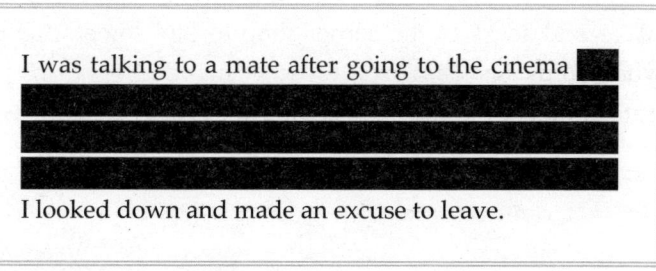

I was talking to a mate after going to the cinema

I looked down and made an excuse to leave.

Read over what you are left with. Hopefully you can see that when we do not base what happened on our self-critical thoughts and feelings the account reads in quite a different way. What a camera would have seen would have been rather different.

Embracing 'mistakes'

If there were no 'mistakes' in the world there would be no learning. The world's first car ever built had no brakes/ gears, couldn't get up a hill and repeatedly crashed. It was the many mistakes that led to the invention of car brakes and gears.

So rather than putting yourself down when something goes wrong, could you try reminding yourself that 'mistakes' are just a part of learning? This is easier said than done if you are used to being hard on yourself when something doesn't go to plan or if others around you can be critical. To get some practice you might want to try getting a few small things wrong on purpose.

Wear odd socks to the corner shop to buy something; get your words mixed up on purpose when ordering a drink in a café; drop your keys when waiting at the bus stop.

Look around and notice how others respond, but also use this as a chance to speak to yourself as you would to your good friend. Embrace the mistake – *This is a sign I'm human! All humans make mistakes; it is the only way we grow and learn.*

Elyse's reflections

I felt like I always had to get things right. The marking scheme I was grading myself on was much harsher than the one I was using for other people. I had to realise that's not fair to me. That's putting me at a disadvantage. I'm always going to come out worse in my head if I'm using a harsher scale. By deliberately slipping on my words or telling a wrong 'fact' I was able to discover that these things do not matter.

Key points and giving myself credit (with kindness!)

 Well done for finishing this chapter. We have covered a lot. Let's pause now and think about what you can give yourself credit for. Remember, ignore that inner critic and think about what you would say to a good friend.

Read Nita's example:

What I can give myself credit for	Key learning points
Reading the chapter. Practising speaking to myself like I would to a friend. Tuning away from the critic and into what others might really be thinking. Be kind, rewind. Embracing mistakes – I was brave and tried making a few small mistakes on purpose.	• Self-criticism is common. • It is also unhelpful and fuels social anxiety. • Time to start noticing when I'm putting myself down. • Give my inner critic a name and remind myself 'it's the critic and not what others are thinking'. • Writing down what I would say to a friend and saying these things to myself helped. • People have around 6,000 thoughts a day. • Drawing out all the kinds of things others think helped me see that the thing I was worried about was less significant to them. • Rewinding what happened and removing my critical thoughts helps me see the facts, not what I imagined. • When I made mistakes, it wasn't a big deal. Nobody responded badly. Mistakes are human.

Now it's your turn:

What I can give myself credit for	Key learning points

Chapter 9

Other People and Me – Building Closer Relationships

Now that you are getting out of your head (Chapter 3) and doing confidence experiments (introduced in Chapter 5) we hope you are feeling less anxious in social situations and more connected with other people. But you might still be finding your friendships challenging. Perhaps you are struggling with the idea of an intimate relationship.

This chapter is all about:

- How social anxiety can affect our friendships and close relationships

- What we can do to improve our connections

Teenage relationships are tough for everyone!

We are social animals. We live, study and work with other people. Our everyday lives depend on a web of social networks.

Why is that? Well, it is nothing new: connecting with other people and helping one another was probably the key to our survival and success as a species! In the days of hunter-gathering, information about food sources or dangers could be shared among individuals and groups. If a member of a group was sick, they could be nursed back to health by the others. It gave us the edge in the fight to survive, and it still does.

So we are built to seek out relationships. But you might have noticed that relationships feel more important at the moment than when you were in primary school. That's because adolescence is the time when we learn about relationships. We spend more time with people the same age as us (our peer group) than at any other point in our lives. We are becoming increasingly independent from our parents (even if they are still nagging you about your messy bedroom!). Adolescence is the time that we learn about relationships so we are set up for adult life. And for everyone there are some things that go wrong in their relationships. There will be bumps in the road; that is part of learning. Working through the ups and downs of relationships in adolescence readies us to become adults.

But it can be tough – sometimes we are thrown together with people we might not have chosen to be our friends. Perhaps you look around and feel like everyone else has their gang of friends, but you don't. It can feel really worrying if you feel like you haven't found your tribe yet. But there are so many people in the world that you are going to cross paths with and that you will have the chance to connect with. Right now, even if you don't connect with the people in your class, try to view your interactions with your peers as opportunities. They are opportunities to learn skills for later life.

So, our relationships often feel a top priority in adolescence. This means that teenagers tend to be on high alert for all things friendship-related. And so most of us feel an uptick in social fears when we become teenagers – it is really normal.

Here are some other examples:

- Teenagers in general tend to worry about relationships more than at any other time in life. We think this is because relationships are so important at this time of our lives. This means that all of us as teenagers tend to be concerned about being invited to things and being liked by other people.

- Compared to kids and adults, teenagers get a bigger rush of happiness from positive social experiences and a bigger hit of sadness from negative ones. This means that teenagers in general tend to be more sensitive to being slighted or pushed away by others.

- We get more self-conscious when we are teenagers – we are really aware of how we think we come across to others, what other people might be thinking of us. This means that all of us as teenagers tend to feel like we are the centre of others' attention.

- Our decisions are more influenced by what other teenagers think when we are teenagers. When we are kids and adults, the decisions we make are similar whether we're on our own, with people our own age or with people of a different age. When we are teenagers, we are more willing to take risks when we are with other teenagers than when we are alone or with kids or adults. This means that teenagers may do things when they are with their peers that they wouldn't do otherwise, and this can include making bad calls, such as trying something risky or dangerous or joining in with teasing or bullying someone.

Is this surprising? Lots of young people tell us that they thought they were the only ones who felt self-conscious. The only one who felt worried about their relationships. Although people vary, and of course there are some super-confident people, most teenagers are experiencing at least a degree of what you are feeling too. You are not alone. It also helps explain why relationships can feel so difficult when we're teenagers – it is because **everyone** is worrying about whether they have upset someone, whether they will be included in a group, whether everyone is looking at them, and because everyone is experiencing strong emotions in their relationships.

Social anxiety and friendship difficulties: chicken or egg?

Imagine this . . .

You text a group of friends and suggest meeting up at the weekend. One of your friends explains she can't make it because she has too much work to do.

OK, that's understandable – we all have weekends when we're behind on work, right?

The same group of friends suggests meeting up another weekend. That same person says again she can't make it.

And the same the next time.

Hmm, now what are you thinking? Maybe something is up with her?

You ask, but she says nothing is the matter.

What do you take from that? Do you start wondering whether she is just not interested in hanging out with you? That she would prefer to do something else?

What might you do next time you meet up with friends?

You would be forgiven for not including the person in the invite.

You might just assume she would turn you down.

But here's the kicker – what if this person is really socially anxious and keeps turning you down because although she'd love to be friends with you, she fears you're only inviting her to be polite, that you don't really want her there?

Social anxiety can lead us to act in ways that send the opposite message to the one we intended. In the rest of this chapter, we are going to look at how social anxiety affects our relationships and what we can do about it.

Before we think about how social anxiety affects our friendships and romantic relationships, let's take a moment to think about the other side of the coin – how difficult experiences with other people can impact social confidence.

Those who experience more difficult experiences with other people – like being rejected or bullied – tend to go on to experience more social anxiety over time. We know this from research we have done at the University of Oxford.

You may recognise this yourself and remember reading about it in Chapter 1. Perhaps you experienced challenging times in your friendship or relationships that you feel contributed to you losing social confidence.

Our experiences affect how we see ourselves and other people; if the experiences are negative – a friend dropping you, being treated badly by someone at school – it can lead us to see ourselves as unacceptable or unlikeable more generally.

We hope that you have been learning through this book that this is **not** true! When you don't hide away and you give people a chance to know you, people will accept you just as you are. If somebody behaved in an unpleasant or unkind way towards you, it says more about them than it does about you. Take a look at Chapter 11, which is all about bullying in the past and present.

OK, let's get back to thinking about the flip side of the coin.

We can all fall into the trap of assuming that everyone else is super-confident and socially savvy, and it is only us that has self-doubt, anxieties and hang-ups. But this isn't true. All of us have fears, quirks and vulnerabilities, and we bring this baggage to our friendships. And so friendships work best when we are clear to the other person that we like them, that we accept them and want to spend time with them. The problem with social anxiety is that it can make it hard to do this. Even though we might really want to form a friendship and connect with someone, somehow we give off a different signal. And then what happens is that the other person follows the script.

Let's learn about ways social fears can affect how we respond and relate to other people, because if we can spot these then perhaps we can interrupt the cycle.

Elyse's reflections

It took a while to realise that I was isolating myself and I needed to try not to shut myself away. I wouldn't text people, so people wouldn't text me back. I assumed people didn't invite me out because they didn't want to hang out with me. It took me a while to realise that I wasn't putting the effort into the relationships either. I was giving the message that I didn't want to hang out. But when I started initiating things more, then I got invited along more. People realised that I did want to go to things, and this in turn would help foster the relationship. I've learnt we share responsibility for our relationships. If you're not putting the effort in yourself, it's not going to pay back.

Missing the moments

When we avoid social situations because of anxiety, it gives us short-term relief, but we miss out on opportunities to forge friendships.

How do I avoid situations?

❑ Make an excuse to leave early

❑ Turn down invitations

❑ Only attend social events accompanied by close friends

❑ Stay silent on a messaging group

❑ Don't reply to messages

❑ Avoid arranging social events/inviting people

❑ Screen calls

For example, after football practice most people hung around and chatted for a while, but Josh would make excuses and leave as soon as it finished. This is because he was worried people would find him boring. The weekly practice became more and more awkward for Josh. He continued to believe he was boring and that people didn't want to speak to him. But as well as this, the rest of the team got closer to one another, they became mates and started organising socials. This left Josh feeling out on a limb and separate.

What we can see in Josh's example is that avoiding other people prevented him from testing out his fears but also meant he missed out on the opportunity to get to know them. This left him feeling lonely and isolated from the group.

Let's take a moment to map out what happens.

Here is what Josh mapped out:

Thought:	They'll find me boring
Situation I avoid:	The post-footy chat
Effect on:	
Thought:	Still convinced they'll find me boring
Relationships:	They're getting closer and I still feel like a stranger
Loneliness/ connection:	Feeling less connected to the others week by week

If you ticked 'yes' to ways of avoiding situations above, then it's your turn:

Thought: _____

Situation I avoid: _____

Effect on:

Thought: _____

_____

Relationships: _____

_____

Loneliness/
connection: _____

_____

Now it's time to start CATCHING the moment

The good thing here is that you already know what to do to start catching the moment: confidence experiments! But if you have been missing the moment for a while, then it can take a bit longer to see what happens to our relationships when we start catching the moment. Relationships don't change overnight.

We can find out what happened with Josh when he started catching the moment:

👣 Step 1. Belief	👣 Step 2. Situation	👣 Step 3. Predict	👣 Step 4. Do it!	👣 Step 5. Reflect	👣 Step 6. Look ahead
I'm boring.	Post-footy chat.	They will all chat, I will be on the edge and they won't include me. I'll have nothing to say – 75%.	Stay after footy on a regular basis. Drop behaviour traps and keep my attention on the others.	I stayed for the chat every week. No one excluded me. To begin with, I felt like I wasn't 'in the loop' with the topics of conversation and that felt a little awkward. But I reminded myself that it is no surprise that I wasn't in the loop – I hadn't been there and they had chatted every week. I stuck with it, got to know the others and over time I was 'in the loop'. Belief now – 20%.	If I give people a chance to include me, they will. I've noticed I do this in school as well. Like I tend to avoid going to the lunch hall. I'm going to start doing that and see what happens when I join the others.

Why don't you have a go now?

Step 1. Belief	Step 2. Situation	Step 3. Predict	Step 4. Do it!	Step 5. Reflect	Step 6. Look ahead	
What fearful belief will you focus on?	*What situation will you test out your fear in?*	*What is the worst that you think might happen?* *How would you know?* *0–100%*	*How will you test it out?* *Remember to get externally focused and drop behaviour traps.*	*What happened?* *Re-rate your prediction (0–100%).* *What does this tell you about yourself more generally?*	*What are you going to try next to build on your learning?*	

Sending the wrong message

We have learnt that when we feel anxious in social situations, when we worry about messing up and being judged, we tend to fall into behaviour traps. We think these help keep us safe from messing up, but we have discovered in this book that they backfire.

They backfire because they prevent us from discovering our fears are not going to happen anyway. But behaviour traps cause other problems too. They can get in the way of our relationships. Let's take a closer look.

The girl who sits next to Nita in tutor time, Sarah, is really nice. But because Nita worries about blushing, she tends to avoid eye contact and keep quiet when Sarah tries to strike up a conversation. Nita has noticed that Sarah is making less effort with her recently.

Why is this? Why is Sarah cooling off Nita? If we take a moment to think about how Nita's classmate might feel, then it's perhaps no surprise. When we don't make eye contact and don't engage in conversation it sends a message to the other person. The message is: *I'm not interested!* Now of course **we** know that Nita is interested. She wants nothing more than to connect with people. But her behaviour traps are giving off a very different message. And remember, other teenagers, like Sarah, are worried about being rejected too. So they are looking out for the friendship green lights and are quick to back off if they see a warning signal.

Have a think about your interactions. Do you do any of the following?

❏ Avoid eye contact

❏ Hold back from saying things

❏ Speak quietly

❏ Don't ask questions

❏ Give short answers

❏ Draw conversations to a close as quickly as possible

❏ Find an excuse to leave a situation

❏ Check your phone frequently so you aren't drawn into a conversation

❏ Be irritable/short with other people

❏ Any others

Behaviour trap	Why I do it	What effect does it have on my belief?	What unhelpful signal could it give off to other people?

Now it's time to start GIVING THE GREEN LIGHT

We will use confidence experiments here but there are a few things to bear in mind.

- We cannot expect other people to catch on straight away to the different signals you are sending. You will need to persist with the confidence experiments over days and weeks and remain on the lookout for how others are responding to you to see the change in action.

- It can be a good idea to start off your confidence experiments with people in a new setting (such as a club, group or workplace outside school) or in a one-to-one setting with a classmate in school. This is because if you have been socially anxious for a while, you might find that you and your peers have got stuck in a negative rut. Perhaps some of your classmates are not friendly to you. This can make it difficult to do confidence experiments with some people, particularly in the beginning.

We can find out what happened with Nita when she started giving the green light:

🐾 Step 1. Belief	🐾 Step 2. Situation	🐾 Step 3. Predict	🐾 Step 4. Do it!	🐾 Step 5. Reflect	🐾 Step 6. Look ahead
I blush.	In class with Sarah.	She will notice I'm going red and think I'm a nervous mess and not want to talk to me – 60%.	Chat to Sarah, make eye contact and ask her questions. Do this every day in tutor time.	I chatted to Sarah every day in tutor time. To start with, Sarah was nice but it felt like she held back a bit. Although I was worried, I told myself to stick with it and I kept chatting to her every day. Sarah and I started clicking as we chatted more. I learnt that my fears were wrong and Sarah is now beginning to feel like a friend. Belief now – 20%.	I'm going to join Sarah and her friends to walk home after school – and remember to give the green light to them too.

Ready to have a go?

Take a look at the behaviour traps you ticked. Which one will you focus on first?

Step 1. Belief	Step 2. Situation	Step 3. Predict	Step 4. Do it!	Step 5. Reflect	Step 6. Look ahead
What fearful belief will you focus on?	What situation will you test out your fear in?	What is the worst that you think might happen? How would you know? 0–100%	How will you test it out? Remember to get externally focused and drop behaviour traps.	What happened? Re-rate your prediction (0–100%). What does this tell you about yourself more generally?	What are you going to try next to build on your learning?

Being the servant

People with social anxiety often find it hard to stand up for themselves, to say what they want or express their preferences and wishes. This can be because of a fear that others will be angry with them or that other people only tolerate them because they fit in and do as they are asked.

Do you do any of the following?

❑ Say yes to things that you don't really want to do

❑ Put your own needs second

❑ Go out of your way to please others

❑ Avoid saying no to people

❑ Avoid sharing your problems and difficulties

It is really understandable if you do, but as we have learnt these behaviours prevent us from testing out our fears. How can you discover that it is OK to say 'no' without trying it out?

But also, these behaviour traps can get in the way of developing a genuine connection with someone. Proper friendship happens when we really know one another:

• It is brilliant to celebrate our friends' successes, but it is just as important to share their upsets and struggles. It is often in the sharing of difficulties that even closer bonds are formed. It allows the other person to feel able to share their difficulties, to feel like they know the person better and to feel trusted.

- Being the servant can mean a friendship is unbalanced and leave you feeling unsupported and undervalued.

True friendships are based on a balance of give and take.

Time for some detective work:

Let's begin by learning from others. When you're with other people – this might be a group of people you hang out with or a group of people you are sitting within earshot of – listen to their conversation and ask yourself the following questions:

- How are decisions (about what to do, where to go) reached?

- What happens if someone says 'no' to a request?

Discoveries and reflections: Take a moment to note down what you learnt from this exercise. What does it suggest about give and take in friendships? Is it OK to say no?

Now it's time to 'back yourself'

You are now ready to take the next step and try a confidence experiment. If you tend to avoid saying 'no' to people, then try saying 'no' next time. Remember to keep your attention focused on the outside and drop those behaviour traps (which might include making sure you don't apologise after you've said 'no', avoiding eye contact, speaking quietly). If you tend to agree with other people, try expressing your opinion if it differs from others. And if you tend not to share your problems with others, then when something has upset you, try sharing it with someone you trust. Start with sharing a small problem if you find it hard to begin with.

Step 1. Belief	Step 2. Situation	Step 3. Predict	Step 4. Do it!	Step 5. Reflect	Step 6. Look ahead
What fearful belief will you focus on?	What situation will you test out your fear in?	What is the worst that you think might happen? How would you know? 0–100%	How will you test it out? Remember to get externally focused and drop behaviour traps.	What happened? Re-rate your prediction (0–100%). What does this tell you about yourself more generally?	What are you going to try next to build on your learning?

Sticking with the herd

Fears that we'll look foolish or get it wrong can make us want to hide our own tastes and follow other people's instead to blend in – we 'follow the herd'.

This can backfire because we don't get the chance to express ourselves fully or give others the space to do that themselves. Common interests are great, but points of difference are just as important in a friendship. It wouldn't be very interesting if our friends had exactly the same tastes and opinions as us!

What are the possible benefits of expressing your own tastes and preferences? Take a moment to think about your favourite musicians, artists, designers or video game developers. What made them special? Now think about your close friends or family members. What is it that you like most about them? Most likely, what is special about those artists and most lovable in those closest to you are the things that are unique to them. Their different take on the world, surprising tastes and fresh perspective. It would be quite a dull world if we all thought the same thing.

Now it's time to express yourself!

Let's look at what Nita did. Nita tended to wear plain, dark clothes by brands that she knew her friends wore. She didn't want to draw attention to herself or to stand out. But Nita loved clothes and fashion. She had some items in her wardrobe that were bright and bold. She would love to wear them but instead they stayed in her cupboard because she feared the reaction she would get if she wore them out. She decided she would do her first confidence experiment by expressing herself with her clothes. She went into town to meet a friend on a Saturday morning and wore a bright top. She made sure not to cover it up and to keep her attention on those around her, to see how they reacted to her. It was an eye-opening experience! Not only did no one give her unfriendly looks as she had feared, but her friend gave her a compliment. From this confidence experiment, Nita pressed on with many more, expressing herself through clothes, music choices and sharing her opinions.

What 'expressing yourself' confidence experiment will you start with? Remember to drop your behaviour traps and get out of your head. Good luck!

👣 Step 1. Belief	👣 Step 2. Situation	👣 Step 3. Predict	👣 Step 4. Do it!	👣 Step 5. Reflect	👣 Step 6. Look ahead						
What fearful belief will you focus on?	*What situation will you test out your fear in?*	*What is the worst that you think might happen?* *How would you know?* *0–100%*	*How will you test it out?* *Remember to get externally focused and drop behaviour traps.*	*What happened?* *Re-rate your prediction (0–100%).* *What does this tell you about yourself more generally?*	*What are you going to try next to build on your learning?*						

Misreading the moment

Reading social situations is hard. People's meanings, intentions and reactions are rarely 100% clear. We have to do a lot of interpreting of what people say and do to understand their meaning. Sarcasm can be the hardest – is the person teasing us playfully or do they really mean it? Is it a compliment or a jibe? Feeling socially anxious can make it even harder to work out what people mean. That is because when we feel socially anxious, we tend to read the room negatively. For example, someone misses an easy cross in football and a teammate calls out, 'Nice one, slowcoach!' Or a student gets three answers right in a row in class and a classmate says, 'Ooh, show off!'

It can be hard to know. If you are frequently the butt of the joke and you feel upset by it, then have a look at Chapter 11, Dealing with Bullies or Teasing (in the Past or Present). But sometimes, when we are socially anxious, we can react to a playful tease in a way that backfires. We can misread a friendly joke as something unkind. And then because we react as if the person was being mean, it can put a wedge in that relationship. Let's take a closer look.

> Two classmates, Tiana and Clare, are waiting for the lesson to start. They are talking and comparing their homework. Clare says, 'That's funny, we wrote the same explanation for that answer!' and Tiana replies, 'That's because you're *always* copying over my shoulder.'

Clare can read this in two ways and both interpretations pop into her mind. One interpretation is that it is a playful tease: neither she nor Tiana believes Clare copies. Another interpretation is that Tiana actually finds Clare annoying and maybe she does think she copies her work (even if Clare knows that she doesn't). She has to choose which interpretation to go with.

If Clare reads this as a playful tease, she could react in a few ways. She could smile and the conversation moves on. She could react with a gentle joke back – 'Exactly, so where's this week's science homework for me to copy now?!' – which Tiana laughs at.

If Clare reads this as an accusation, she would react differently. She might look away and go silent. She might turn back to her work. She might become upset or annoyed.

Think for a moment about how the interaction might go differently depending on which interpretation Clare goes with . . .

When we see ourselves in a negative way, it can make us quick to interpret other people's comments in a negative way too. Look back over the past few weeks and jot down one or two examples of when people have made comments to you that you were uncertain about. Comments that perhaps you felt a bit hurt or offended by but you weren't sure if you overreacted. As you read the comments ask yourself:

- Does that person make similar comments to other people?

- How would I react if that person made the same comment to someone else?

- How has that person reacted to me every day since?

- Am I taking that too personally?

- Am I jumping to conclusions?

- Is my inner critic doing the talking?

- Is there another way of thinking about it?

Now you have had a chance to consider the comments in this new way, what conclusions can you draw? If it feels like you are repeatedly being targeted with unkind comments, then go to Chapter 11, Dealing with Bullies or Teasing (in the Past or Present).

But if you are spotting that you have interpreted the comments through the lens of your negative view of yourself then it is time to try responding to these kinds of comments differently. Test out reacting to them as if they are meant as well-intentioned jokes rather than mean insults and check out the result.

Moth to the flame

Why do we have the friends we do?

Hopefully our friends are people:

- We share interests and values with

- We like spending time with

- Who make us laugh

- We feel we can turn to for support or help

Sometimes social anxiety can affect the choices we make about who we spend our time with. When we feel uncertain if we will be accepted by other people, and unsure of ourselves, it can be tempting to seek out approval from those people who seem confident, sorted and strong. If those people let you hang out with them, it can feel like a seal of approval, a sign you have 'passed' somehow, that maybe you are acceptable. It is a bit like a moth being drawn to a flame over and over, even though it might hurt them.

In Nita's year at school there was a big group of girls. They were the popular girls, the girls who made the most noise and seemed to dominate the classroom. Nita hung out on the fringes of the group. She hoped she might be allowed to join their table at lunchtime, their group text calls and out-of-school meetings. But this didn't always happen; sometimes she would be allowed to join them but other times she would be left out. She never quite felt like she fitted in with them. Somehow hanging out with them never made her feel OK about herself, because even if she joined the girls at lunch one day, she was never sure she would be let in the next day. And she couldn't shake a nagging feeling that she didn't really fit in with them. She wasn't one of them.

What was going on for Nita? To understand it, let's take a step back. Nita took some time to think about what she really wanted in a friend. This is what she came up with:

What I look for in a friend:

- Kindness and loyalty
- Similar sense of humour
- Likes fashion design, sewing, music, cooking
- Feels good when I'm with them

Nita then thought about the girls she was hanging out with and how they matched up with the list of things that mattered to her in a friend. There was some overlap – like interest in fashion and music – but Nita noticed that this group didn't find the same things funny, they didn't care about design and making (Nita's passion) or cooking. And most importantly, she didn't feel cared for with this group of people.

If you think you might be in a similar situation to Nita, why don't you start by jotting down your thoughts about what you really want in a friend?

Now reflect on how the people you hang out with at the moment fit the list. Most importantly, are they kind people?

Finding your people

So, what to do now? You might have decided that the people you're hanging out with now are OK but that it's time to spark some new friendships. In the past, this was probably difficult to do because you felt socially anxious. But with this book you will have come a long way in building your confidence and you are now ready to seek out new connections. The new connections might be with people you come across day to day who perhaps you've overlooked up to now. Or it might be about creating new opportunities to meet people, like joining a club or group linked to one of your passions. Remember – confidence experiments will help you to do this!

Nita made a start by doing confidence experiments with a girl in her tutor group in school and by joining a dressmaking class on Saturdays.

Key points and giving yourself credit

 Well done. We have covered a lot. Let's take a moment to give yourself credit.

Josh's example:

What I can give myself credit for	Key learning points
Reading through the chapter and understanding how social anxiety can interfere with my friendships.	• Social anxiety can get in the way of my relationships. • Look out for how my social anxiety is interfering. • I sometimes misread what friends are saying. If friends banter, I can take it too much to heart. I will try to laugh next time and get involved in the chat rather than leaving the room and taking it too personally. • I can plan some confidence tasks to speak up more around the others in my film class. I know I have lots in common with others there and it would be good for them to get to know me more.

Now it's your turn:

What I can give myself credit for	Key learning points

Chapter 10

Social Media and Me

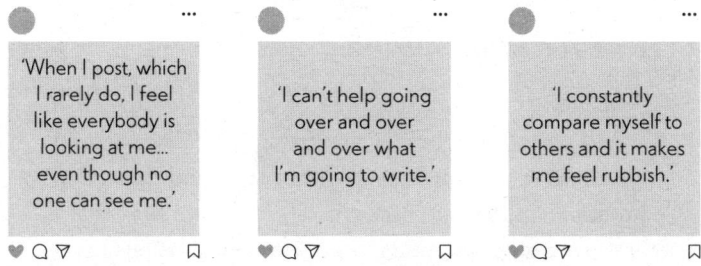

'When I post, which I rarely do, I feel like everybody is looking at me... even though no one can see me.'

'I can't help going over and over and over what I'm going to write.'

'I constantly compare myself to others and it makes me feel rubbish.'

Does any of this sound familiar? If so, you are not alone. These are quotes taken from interviews we did with socially anxious people about their life on social media. For many people the online world is not an escape from social anxiety.

As social media can feel less intense than coming face to face with someone, it could be a place that we build our confidence gradually. But instead, when our social fears pop up online, it drains our confidence. We often fall into the same old behaviour traps that keep us stuck feeling anxious: holding back, rarely posting, overthinking everything we share. So how can we use the online world to feel more connected, rather than lonely and anxious? Let's find out.

This chapter is about:

- Stepping away from comparing ourselves to others online

- Learning to be authentic online without overthinking it

- Being kind to yourself online

Elyse's reflections

Social media was a big area of anxiety for me. If a friend posted a picture of me that I didn't like, I would obsess over it, look over it and over it, find flaws and I'd ask them to take it down. The problem was that I was spending so much time looking at a post that I would assume that everyone else was doing the same. But most people look at a post for no more than thirty seconds and it's forgotten within another thirty seconds, because most people don't tend to remember things that don't directly involve them.

Is social media your friend or your enemy?

The aim of social media is to build our connections – but, for many, it feels less like a friendly space and more like somewhere else we just don't fit in. Why is this? This can be a result of the behaviour traps we understandably fall into using online. Look at the list below and tick any that apply to you:

When online I . . .

❑ Compare myself unfairly to others

❑ Put myself down

❑ Don't share myself

❑ Spend lots of time preparing what to share

❑ Overthink what I add

❑ Monitor how many likes or responses I get

❑ Watch myself rather than others

❑ Spend too much time scrolling

Lots of people feel some anxiety on social media and under-standably do some of the above. But what is the impact? We end up feeling lonely, cut off and more anxious. We miss get-ting anything positive from being online. To start enjoying social media more, the key is to escape from some of these traps. Let's find out how.

Stop comparing yourself

Josh found himself looking at his friends' photos and posts over the holidays. He felt like everybody was hav-ing more fun than he was. He thought, Why am I so

> *dull? He felt boring and low. What Josh did not see was*
> *all the moments his friends had also felt bored over the*
> *holidays too. He just saw the brief, fun moments they*
> *chose to post.*

Spending even a few minutes comparing yourself to others online can leave you feeling badly about yourself. This is because it is an unfair comparison.

Here are two key reasons why:

1. **You cannot see the full picture.** You know yourself inside out: your highs and lows, all the flaws and blemishes that make you wonderfully human. But when looking at somebody else's post or profile you see only what they have chosen to share, which is a tiny fraction of the whole person.

   Imagine holding a piece of paper in front of your face to block your vision, then making a tiny pinhole through it. If you were to examine somebody else's life by looking through that tiny hole you might make out the odd thing but miss 99% of what is happening. This is what it is like scrolling through someone's posts. If somebody shares a photo of themselves smiling at a party, what you do not see is the row they had with their mum or dad just before, the moments they felt down about themselves that night.

2. **Real life is hidden behind the filters.** Many people try hard to make themselves and their lives look better online. The human flaws and blemishes we all have that

might be spotted in person are often hidden. If you follow online influencers, remember that social media may be a full-time job for them. They spend huge amounts of time and resources to get things to look a certain way. Well-lit, airbrushed shots and scripted videos are not real life. Real life is imperfect. It is a messy bedroom, a falling-out with a friend or family member, a moment of anger or irritability.

So, try not to compare yourself to the airbrushed snaps you see online. It is an unfair comparison.

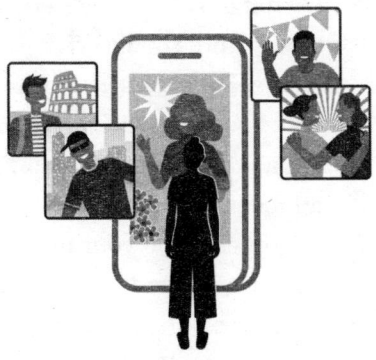

It might also help to follow a range of people. Some people are more likely to share more 'real' content than others. Try following some people who share more of life's challenges, the downs as well as the ups, shots without make-up, etc.

Try to be aware of spending too much time scrolling, too, as this can affect your mood. It is helpful to get a balance of activities in your life. Be sure to plan time to exercise and do other things you enjoy offline to help manage your mood.

To share or not to share?

When feeling anxious online, we tend to hold back, to watch what others do and share less of ourselves. If we share, we might overthink what to say and monitor the reactions too closely. These behaviour traps have the same impact online as they do in person: they can make us feel cut off and unaccepted by others.

 **Here are some tips on sharing online:**

★ **Do not overthink it.** Everybody thinks a little about what they share online. But unless you make a career out of being on social media, sharing online should not be a full-time commitment. Trying to perfect a photo or post eats into your time, drives up your anxiety and steals the joy from using social media. To give you an idea about what your peers are doing, it might help to ask a trusted friend how much time they spend thinking about things they share. Helpful questions you could ask might include:

  ° How often do you post something on x/y platform?

° When you post something, how much time do you spend thinking about it beforehand?

You might then want to treat it as a confidence experiment to try sharing something without excessively checking it or censoring it. Think about what you would tell a good friend to do if they were holding back so much. Try to take your own good advice!

★ **Let it go! Let it go!** Once you post something, try not to keep checking how many thumbs-up or emojis it gets. This does not relate to your worth and often has more to do with the amount of online noise at the time. Overly focusing on something you have posted will give you a false sense that other people are scrutinising it too – but are they?

The stats on the amount people post online are constantly increasing, but google it yourself and you will be shocked by how many millions of photos and posts are shared each minute on different platforms. It might help to remember that your post is one of millions made that day. So, if it has not had the response you were hoping for, others may not have registered it or have simply moved on with their day. Sharing online can feel like you have just shouted something out in the middle of a quiet lecture hall, and everybody is staring at you. It is more like whispering something during a gig that is drowned out by the noise. It can help to remind yourself of this. Bringing to mind an image that illustrates this might help if you are finding yourself worrying about a post; for example, picturing your post like a tiny grain of sand on miles of beach.

To help with this, you could google 'Erik Kessels' Flickr exhibition'. This artist printed images shared over twenty-four hours on one social media site back in 2011. Looking at the sea of photos in his exhibition gives you an idea of how much content is shared each day (and 2011 was a good few years ago!).

Josh shared a photo of himself online with his new dog. He found afterwards he was overthinking his post and monitoring how many people commented or liked it. He was getting more and more anxious about it. After a while he tried instead to remind himself that there are millions of photos shared every minute online. He pictured his photo like one grain of sand on a mile of beach to help keep this in perspective. When he saw his friends the next day nobody brought it up. It wasn't headline news to them; it was just another post among many hundreds they scrolled through. Some hadn't even seen it.

Focus on others, not yourself

Much like when you are talking to somebody in person, if you are chatting via text or video call, it is still important to watch out for times when you start overly focusing on yourself and how you are coming across. Remember what we covered in Chapter 3, Getting out of My Head and Enjoying Social Situations – focus instead on the other person. Look at their video, not your own. Tune in to what they are saying in their messages, rather than focusing too much on yourself and what you are going to say next or looking over messages you have just written. Get interested in other people rather than focusing on yourself.

If you find this hard during a video chat, it might help to hide your own image, so that you can only see the other person. This may help you focus more on them, rather than on yourself. Or just try glancing briefly at yourself in a kinder way – to remind yourself that you look just like any other person on a webchat.

Be kind to yourself online

When online – whether scrolling or sharing – our inner critic can often pop up. 'They are having more fun than you are', 'You don't have anything funny or interesting to say', 'You shouldn't have shared that, you idiot'. You would never dream of speaking to a good friend like this – it would make them feel awful! So keep your eye out for when the inner critic gets going. This is your chance to tune in to what you would be saying to a friend or loved one instead. You might find it helpful to review Chapter 8, Be Kind to Myself, if you find this hard. It can take a bit of practice.

Below are some examples of the kinds of things that Josh tried saying to himself when his inner critic started talking:

Self-critical thought online	Kinder response I would say to a friend
They are having more fun than you.	You are only seeing a tiny fraction of what they chose to share.
You don't have anything funny or interesting to say.	It's not my job to entertain people online. I'm not an online comedian. Not everybody posts funny and fascinating things all the time – that's not real life.
You shouldn't have shared that, you idiot.	Well done for sharing something when you don't usually do it much. Now try to get on with something else today. Don't overthink it.

You might want to make a note of some of your common self-critical thoughts online and note down some of your own kinder responses. It might help to have these written somewhere to hand or saved on your phone.

Self–critical thought online	Kinder response I would say to a friend

Take action

Confidence tasks to try online

 If you have worked through the chapter on particular fears, you might already have some ideas of the kinds of confidence tasks that might test out some of the fears you have online. The kinds of things you could try might include:

- Texting with some friends without overly preparing your responses

- Sharing something online without overthinking it beforehand or afterwards

- Liking or responding to a post rather than reading it and staying quiet

---

Elyse's reflections

What would I tell you now I've overcome my social media anxiety? Just don't dwell on it. People are constantly scrolling. They spend ten seconds max looking at a post. They aren't scrutinising it like you are. Now I post what I want to, rather than what I think people want me to post. I post and then I put my phone down. I don't obsess over it. I let go of who is commenting or liking it. I get on with something else.

Below is an example of an experiment Josh did on his phone to test his fear of coming across as boring.

Step 1. Belief	Step 2. Situation	Step 3. Predict	Step 4. Do it!	Step 5. Reflect	Step 6. Look ahead
I'm boring.	Sharing more in a group chat with friends.	I'll come across as boring – 60%. The others will ignore me, not respond at all or kick me out of the group chat.	Rather than staying quiet, respond in the chat if I want without overly planning what I'm going to say.	It was tough at first as nobody responded for a while, but that happens with text – then a couple of people did and I didn't get kicked out of the group. Maybe I'm not as boring as I feel. Re-rated prediction – 35%.	I can keep going with responding more on text. It will build my confidence and help me build better friendships.

Now it's your turn:

Step 1. Belief	Step 2. Situation	Step 3. Predict	Step 4. Do it!	Step 5. Reflect	Step 6. Look ahead	
What fearful belief will you focus on?	*What situation will you test out your fear in?*	*What is the worst that you think might happen?* How would you know? 0–100%	*How will you test it out?* Remember to get externally focused and drop behaviour traps.	*What happened?* Re-rate your prediction (0–100%). *What does this tell you about yourself more generally?*	*What are you going to try next to build on your learning?*	

What did I learn?

Did you try some confidence tasks online? What did you learn? What do you plan to do going forward to continue to build your social confidence?

Spend a few moments making a plan, either here or somewhere handy like on your phone.

My plan to keep building on my social confidence online

Troubleshooting

People's responses

If you shared a funny story with a friend in person you would be able to gauge their reaction to it. Online people's responses can be harder to read. For example, Nita shared something that happened to her at college online and a friend replied, 'Funny story.' Nita found herself worrying if they meant her story was entertaining or weird. Nita was looking at their comment through the lens of her own view of herself. She interpreted it negatively because she often thinks of herself as weird. If you find you are reading too much into somebody's response it might help to ask yourself:

- Am I taking that too personally?

- Am I jumping to conclusions?

- Is my inner critic doing the talking?

- Is there another way of thinking about it?

When Nita did this, she was able to see that she was misreading what her friend had said. She tested this out further by speaking to that friend later at school. The friend responded normally to her and did not even bring up the post.

Some young people have had negative experiences online. When Josh was younger somebody in his class put an unfriendly comment on one of his posts. So how do we manage if this happens? Try asking yourself the following questions:

- Would you want to be friends with somebody who puts others down online or posts negative responses?

- Does that sound like somebody you would like and respect?

- Does their response say more about you or the person posting the negative comment?

Josh found it helpful to remind himself that the guy who posted something unfriendly was not a nice guy and not somebody he wanted in his life. He decided to ignore the comment as it didn't deserve his attention. If this is not just one negative comment but a pattern, you might find it help-ful to look at Chapter 11, Dealing with Bullies or Teasing (in the Past or Present).

Key points and giving yourself credit

Well done for working through this section on social media. Take a moment to give yourself credit for working on this chapter and for any of the confidence tasks you tried. Josh made a note of the more helpful strategies he could try online below:

What I can give myself credit for	Key learning points
Reading this chapter.	• Remind myself I only see a tiny fraction of 'real' life online. • Be kind to myself online. • Follow some people who share things in a more 'real' way. • Share what I want to. • Share something without overly preparing it. • Don't overthink what I share. • Let it go! Don't keep checking my posts. • Focus on others in a text/video chat. • Limit my scrolling time.
Experiment with sharing more of myself over text and online without overly preparing it.	• When I share more over text it leads to a better chat and I feel more included in things. • The more I can do this, the more confident I should feel online.

Now it's your turn:

What I can give myself credit for	Key learning points

We hope by trying some of these, you will discover that the online world can begin to be a more enjoyable place to be and somewhere you can start to build connections and confidence. Good luck!

Chapter 11

Dealing with Bullies or Teasing (in the Past or Present)

In this chapter we are going to learn about:

- How to spot if you're being teased or bullied

- What action you can take

- How to overcome upsetting memories from the past of difficult experiences with other people

Relationships are complicated, subtle and nuanced. People can say one thing but mean another. All of us have done unkind things to other people on occasion. But sometimes we are treated in ways that are unkind or cruel and they have lasting effects. This can include bullying and teasing, for example:

- Being called a name

- Being excluded

- Being mocked

- Being hit

- Your possessions being taken

- Rumours being spread about you

- Being isolated from the rest of the group

Unkind behaviour can happen in school, online and at home, and it can take different forms:

Sometimes people bully or tease others by directly hurting them.

This can be verbal, such as name calling, mocking or teasing, or it can be physical, such as hitting, kicking, punching, things being thrown at you or someone repeatedly kicking the back of your chair.

Sometimes people bully or tease others by excluding them from their friendship or friendship group.

This can be by not inviting someone to events, excluding someone from messaging groups, not allowing someone to join the conversation, not letting them join the group, not sharing the joke or telling them the wrong place or time to meet up.

Sometimes people bully or tease others by damaging their reputation or how they are seen by other people.

This can happen when someone spreads rumours about another person or shares embarrassing information about someone with other people.

Why does bullying or teasing happen?

People who experience bullying or teasing often wonder **why** it is happening. They might assume it is something to do with them – because of something that is wrong with them or different about them. But that's not the case. In fact, it is much more to do with the person doing the bullying.

Elyse's reflections

I haven't experienced bullying but friends of mine have. If you are bullied it is not reflective of anything that you've done. It reflects the bully as a person. It is probably to do with things they have gone through in their life, and that's nothing to do with you.

Why do people bully others? Most often, it is to give themselves a feeling of power or control over others. There are a number of reasons why someone might feel the need to do this. Research suggests that people who bully are more likely to:

- Be experiencing difficulties at home. This might be parents with mental health difficulties, parents with drug or alcohol misuse problems, parents or siblings who fight frequently and aggressively.

- Have unstable friendships or a lack of trust in friendships themselves.

- Have low self-esteem, anxiety or mood problems themselves.

- Struggle to control impulses.

- Find it difficult to manage emotions.

- Have learnt to be mean to get what they want.

People bully to give themselves status and power because they feel inadequate in some way. It can be a misguided way to try to feel accepted and liked by others.

Signs I am being bullied or teased

It can be difficult to know if you are being bullied or teased.

You might feel like something is not right but doubt yourself – *Am I overreacting?* – or you might blame yourself for what is going on – *Is it my fault?*

Ask yourself: *If my friend was being treated in this way, would I think it was acceptable?*

If the answer is 'No', then it shouldn't happen to you either.

Bullying makes people feel anxious and can make life miserable. Lots of people who are bullied or teased feel powerless to stop it. Let's take some time to think about what we can do.

I think I am being bullied now. What can I do about it?

1. Tell someone you trust.

   Being bullied makes people feel isolated and alone. It can feel hard to tell anyone; it can feel scary and over-whelming. But it is the first step in making it stop. Find someone you trust – a friend, teacher, parent, carer, rela-tive, activity leader or health care worker – and tell them.

2. Tell your school.

   Most people are bullied by schoolmates. That means school will need to be part of the plan to stop the bul-lying. By law, every school must have an anti-bullying plan. You might not feel comfortable talking to school on your own. If not, then ask your trusted person to help you. For example, maybe you'd prefer your parents to speak to school on your behalf, or perhaps you'd rather be there along with your parents.

3. Keep a diary of what is happening.

   Dates, places, events. Keeping a simple log of your experiences, focusing on the facts rather than feelings, can be helpful for your school as they develop a plan to tackle the bullying.

4. Take care of yourself.

   Even though bullying behaviour says far more about

the bully than it does about you, it takes its toll on the person being bullied. Try to build positive and fulfilling activities into your daily life, however small, and surround yourself with people who support and care for you. Have a look at Chapter 8, Be Kind to Myself – it is full of advice on how to take care of yourself and reduce self-criticism.

5. Develop new connections.

Chapter 9, Other People and Me, is all about the way social anxiety impacts on our relationships and vice versa. In the chapter you will find out about why difficult relationships can make us feel socially anxious. You will also learn the ways that social anxiety can affect our friendships, as well as ideas on what you can do to break the cycle. It may be that you are drawn to people because they are the 'cool' group, the group you feel you should be accepted by – a bit like getting a 'stamp of approval', even though they don't treat you well. But you deserve to be treated well.

I was bullied in the past and I am finding it hard to get over. What can I do?

The ghost from the past

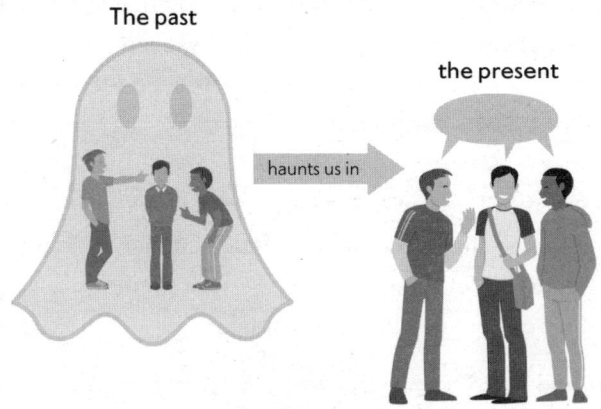

When Josh was eleven or twelve years old, he was picked on by a group of boys at school for the way he looked. As Josh and his peers got a little older this stopped happening. However, whenever Josh was in a group, he often got an uneasy feeling – he felt a little like he did back when he was being bullied. He felt like he was about to be picked on again. Josh was not being bullied, but the memories he had were acting like a ghost from the past, haunting him in the present.

If, like Josh, you find that memories or feelings from past bullying are coming up in the present, we have some tools that can help.

SNAP! Why memories haunt us in the present

Have you ever noticed you hear a particular song playing and suddenly find you are lost in a memory? Without realising why, you find yourself remembering that trip you had to the seaside, when that same song played on repeat in the car. You might even find you start feeling the way you did on that trip. This is because a memory has tumbled out of your memory cupboard. It has fallen into your present. Memory recall is a bit like a game of snap. When you come across something in the present that is similar to something that happened in the past – SNAP! That memory can come tumbling out of your memory cupboard.

So, if you have been bullied or teased in the past and you find yourself in a situation with some similarities, you may start to notice you are feeling some of the feelings you had back then. Josh was bullied by a group of boys when he was eleven. So now when he is in groups – SNAP. He starts to feel as though he will be picked on and ridiculed again. So, what can we do if we notice that a memory/feelings from the past are haunting us in the present? Well, we have a tried-and-tested method we are going to teach you.

Spot the difference!

In our clinic, we have spent many years researching and developing the best ways to help people overcome the impact of traumatic memories. A helpful tool to break the link between the past and present is to play a game of spot the difference. This involves actively looking out for all the things that are different between THEN (the upsetting memory) and NOW (the present). For example, Josh found himself feeling anxious speaking to a group of friends and worrying they would pick on him like others did in the past. He realised these feelings were an echo from his memory. Josh started to spot all the things that were different NOW. He noticed that it was a different time (he was fifteen now, but was eleven back then), it was a different place (he was now in a different form room) and the kids he was speaking to were different too. Importantly, they were not being mean to him now. There was some banter, but this was different from when he was ridiculed in the past.

Spot the Difference

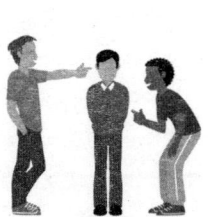 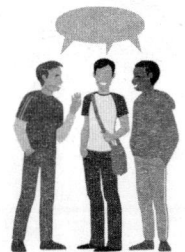

Then

Age 11
Boys were hurting me
Saying mean things
Ridiculing my height

Now

Age 15
Different time/place
I'm taller, they're older
Not hurting me anymore
Sometimes they banter,
but they're not being mean

Think of a time recently when a memory or feelings from your past were triggered. Make a note of the situation. Then, just as Josh did above, write down as many differences as you can between THEN and NOW:

Situation:

Differences between:

THEN (the upsetting memory from my past)	NOW (the present situation)

It can help to save this as a flashcard on your phone or on a card/note to read the next time you are about to go into a similar situation. In the coming week, if you find yourself feeling as though memories from the past are haunting you – try playing spot the difference. Get lost in focusing on all the things that are different NOW.

Key points and giving yourself credit

 Take a moment to think about what you have learnt in this chapter and your next steps.

- What action will you take to get the support and help you need with current bullying?

- What tools could you try out this week (e.g. spot the difference) to help you manage any upsetting memories from the past?

Importantly, coping with bullying – past or present – can be tough. What will you do to take good care of yourself this week? Can you plan some self-care activities? Go to the gym? Do something relaxing, like have a bath or read a book? Do something you enjoy, like watch a favourite film?

Take a moment to note down what you can give yourself credit for and your key learning and action points from this chapter.

Here is what Josh wrote:

What I can give myself credit for	Key learning points
Reading this chapter – it is tough to think about the bullying, but proud of myself for reading this rather than avoiding it. When I was being bullied, I did tell my mum and she spoke to the school. Writing my spot the difference flashcard of all the things that are different NOW. Doing something nice for myself after reading this chapter – I went to the gym and read my book when I got home.	Being bullied is tough to go through. It does happen sometimes but it says more about the other people than it does about me – they are the ones with the problem. Bullies probably feel insecure themselves and may have their own issues and they take it out on others. It is important to tell others if you are being bullied and do things to take good care of yourself and build more positive connections. Memories of bullying from the past can haunt you in the present. If this happens, try to notice when the memories are haunting me and spot all the things that are different now (e.g. different time, place, people).

Now you try:

What I can give myself credit for	Key learning and action points

Chapter 12

Helping Others Help Me

Elyse's reflections

I found it hard to talk to my family about my emotions and what I was going through. Mental health wasn't something we spoke about a lot in the family at the time. For me, there was a negative stigma around mental health in the older generations of my family. It was a hard conversation to start with, but the social anxiety also just made it ten times harder to begin that conversation. But even though it was hard at first, I was so glad I did it. However difficult it feels, I would say – you just need to start that conversation.

This chapter is about how others can help us if we are socially anxious. It includes a guide for family and friends that you might want to share with them.

Shame. Embarrassment. Fear. Like I was revealing some humiliating secret. There never seemed a right point so I kept putting it off. It can be very hard to tell someone you feel socially anxious. But what we have learnt about social anxiety so far is that even when we feel like a ball of anxiety inside, it doesn't show on the outside. We aren't made of glass. So that means your family and friends may not know the reality of what you have been coping with. They might have noticed you have turned down suggestions to do things, you haven't answered the phone, or that you have asked them to put in your order in a café. But because they can't see inside your head or feel your feelings, it is unlikely that they will understand the extent of the worries and stress you have been experiencing. They might not understand the reasons behind your actions. This can lead to frustration on their part, upset on yours, and arguments.

Whether or not you choose to talk about your social anxiety with someone is a personal decision. Many that do choose to talk about it, such as Elyse, find it hugely helpful. Some people choose to talk to their parents; other people choose a relative, close friend or member of school staff. But that is not true for everyone. Some people prefer to manage without talking to others, with the support of books like this.

If you would like to talk about it with someone but you are held back by fears of being judged or feeling ashamed, then take a moment to imagine that your friend or a close relative had been going through what you have recently.

- How would you react if they told you?

- Would you feel glad that they had shared their problem with you?

- Would you think there was something wrong with them? Would you not like them anymore?

- Would you want to support them and help them?

OK, so now flip back to thinking about sharing your social anxiety with a trusted friend or close relative. What are your thoughts now? Do you think you should listen to the inner critic or talk to someone?

Think about:

Who? A parent, relative or close friend – someone you trust.

How? Face to face, on the telephone or via text.

What? If you do want to talk about your social anxiety with a family member or close friend, why not give them some suggestions for how they can help you? You might even give them this book to read. That way they can support you to carry out confidence experiments, keep you motivated and encourage you to set yourself more challenging goals.

Perhaps you don't want them to read the whole book, but you would like your family to understand a bit about what social anxiety is like. Below is a short summary aimed at helping families understand social anxiety and how it can affect people. In the Resources section there is a link that you can send to people so that they can read the information in their own time.

A Family's Guide to Social Anxiety

Elyse's reflections

Elyse is a young person who had social anxiety as a teenager. Here are her thoughts about how she would encourage parents/carers and relatives to support a family member.

As a parent, I would encourage you to be open to whatever your child brings to you. I feel like I probably could have sorted out my social anxiety much sooner if I had felt able to talk to my parents about it earlier.

Some parents may not realise what their child is going through. They may tell them it is not as bad as they think it is. It's important that parents recognise that what the person is feeling is genuine. For parents – it may help to do a little bit of research about social anxiety. It might help you to realise that it's much more common than you know.

Most importantly, you need to be patient with the young person. I think you just have to really be open to listen and not offer solutions all the time. You may want to try to offer a solution, but there isn't always an easy answer. They may want to simply let out feelings that they've been holding in for a long time. Rather than give a solution, I think I would just ask your child what they think you can do for them. What within your power can you do to help them to make them feel better?

What is social anxiety?

Most people feel nervous or uncomfortable in certain social situations. For example, many people tell us that they feel anxious when they have to speak in front of a big audience. Even professional actors and teachers can feel anxious in situations like this. For some people this kind of anxiety and fear can happen in more usual, day-to-day social situations. For example, they might feel anxious having a conversation in a group, it might feel difficult to eat or write in front of other people, to put their hand up in class or to make a comment on social media. People may worry about showing signs of anxiety like shaking, sweating or blushing. These are all examples of social anxiety. People with social anxiety worry about doing badly in social situations or making a fool of themselves in some way.

We see a general increase in social worries as children move into adolescence. You may remember this yourself when you look back to your own teenage years. Friendships are particularly important to teenagers and so it is not surprising that social worries are what preoccupies them. Concerns about being liked, being included, being invited to things and coming across well are all typical. For most teenagers these worries do not get in the way of day-to-day life and they fade over time. But for some teenagers the anxiety becomes a problem. It is more intense and long-lasting, and it interferes with school, relationships and everyday tasks like shopping.

Fears and worries

Different teenagers have different worries when they are in social situations and will feel different anxiety symptoms. Common worries include:

They don't want to be my friend.

I'm boring.

I'm stupid.

They think I'm weird.

I'm unlikeable.

I'll have nothing to say.

It will be awkward.

I'll blush.

I'm shaking.

I'm sweating.

They'll see that I'm anxious.

Everybody is staring at me.

I'm not good enough.

Bodily feelings

Physical symptoms are common, like shaking, sweating, blushing, crying, dizziness, speeded-up heart rate, shaky voice, dry mouth. Other symptoms include difficulty concentrating, getting words wrong, difficulty thinking, mind going blank and so on.

Avoidance

Young people with social anxiety will usually try to avoid or stay away from social situations. This is really understandable because of the anxiety and worry that social situations cause. They might completely avoid some situations, or they might go into social situations but find them really difficult throughout. Anxiety might be triggered by particular things or in a wide range of social situations.

You might notice reluctance to order in a café or to speak to a shop assistant, reluctance to go to school on a speech day, discomfort when being the centre of attention (such as birthdays, photos).

Social anxiety is hard to spot

If it took you a while to realise your child was socially anxious, you are not alone. Many teenagers will not disclose their worries and anxieties even to those closest to them. They will often feel embarrassed and ashamed about their social fears.

What impact can social anxiety have?

Social anxiety can cause problems at home, at school and with friends.

At home, young people might refuse to answer the telephone, to attend family gatherings, or they may remain in their bedroom when guests visit. It can sometimes appear to parents that their child is being defiant in these situations, but we know that in fact it is due to their intense distress.

School life can also be a challenge. Adolescents with social anxiety often find it difficult to concentrate in class because they feel so self-conscious. It is common for young people to avoid participating in class, for example showing reluctance to answer or ask questions, not asking for help or participating in group exercises. Sometimes young people will feel unable to manage going to school at all. Grades are often affected. It can be difficult for parents and teachers to manage these behaviours. Sometimes they are misunderstood as disobedience when in fact they are a sign of intense anxiety and distress.

Friendships are very often affected by social anxiety. Adolescents might turn down invitations, not respond to text or telephone calls, and avoid being with peers at break times in school. As a result, young people with social anxiety can end up losing friends and may sometimes become the victim of teasing and bullying. Young people (whether or not they have social anxiety) are often reluctant to talk to their parents about their friendships and so it can be difficult for parents to know the details of their child's social relationships, including whether they are being bullied.

How can family help?

Do you see your child struggling but they are reluctant to tell you why? This can feel frustrating and make it hard to know how to help. As a result, you and your child can get locked in a cycle of avoidance and arguments. This can end up with both of you feeling demoralised and sad. Parents often end up feeling at a loss. But there are lots of things you can do that can help.

Please keep in mind you will read lots of ideas below which we hope you will find helpful. But, above all else, the most helpful thing you can do is to try to **keep an emotional bond with your child and to keep listening to them**. That means creating pockets of time to be with them, to share the same space (not necessarily having a deep conversation). When do you connect best with your child? At bedtime when you can give them a hug, baking at the weekend, watching sports together, in the car? Keep these windows of connection open.

Catch the criticism

As parents, there is often the temptation to jump into a problem-solving and fixing mode when our child is upset or reluctant to do something. When we can't find an obvious problem (in the café you wonder, *Why **can't** she go up and get some napkins from the counter?*) it can lead to frustration and we can be tempted to tell our child to get on with it or to do it ourselves to save an argument.

In moments like these, try to hold back from snapping at your child or letting your temper show. Catch yourself, hard as it is, because it is likely that your child will be giving themselves a hard time already.

Find the feeling

Once you have caught the criticism, pause. Take a moment to ask yourself how your child might be feeling: *What is going on for them right now?* Is it possible that anxiety is behind their action (or inaction)? For example, *Was she feeling too self-conscious to walk through the café to get the napkins?* Try to find your child's feelings in the moment and then allow your child's feelings (or your sense of your child's feelings) to guide your actions. In the moment, such as in a busy café, that might just be a squeeze of their hand or a warm smile.

Start the conversation

Of course, you will want to help your child overcome their fears, but the moment of high anxiety might not be the moment to start talking about how to manage this. Instead, just log what happened, then when you have some time and space you can reflect on the incident. Does it fit into a pattern in your child's behaviour? What situations tend to spark refusals, upset, avoidance?

It can be hard to start a conversation with your child about your concerns. However much they may want support and guidance, invariably socially anxious children struggle to open up about their difficulties and they may well be resistant to you starting the conversation.

Here are some suggestions for how you might approach a first conversation:

- Pick your moment and go gently

- Use phrases like 'maybe' and 'I wonder' to help your child open up without telling them how they feel

- Convey a sense of understanding that your child's reactions make sense, given their fears

- Validate their feelings

- Be curious

- Remind them that many people have similar fears, and that they are not alone. Sometimes it can be helpful to bring in your own experiences of social anxiety, or that of friends/family, such as anxiety about public speaking

For example: *When we were in the café today, it seemed tricky for you to get the napkins from the counter. Is that right? I wondered whether doing things in front of people is hard for you? Like when we're late for school or when you have to give a talk in class. Lots of people find these sorts of things stressful – they worry about messing up or making a fool of themselves. When I was younger, I used to get really anxious speaking in front of the class because I worried I would mess up my words.*

Be patient; it may well be a slow process. You might find that rather than one in-depth conversation you have a series of brief chats. Keep channels of communication open.

Ask your child how you can help in moments when they feel anxious. What would **they** like you to do to support them to feel more confident? As a parent, your role is to support your child, but you can't dictate the pace.

For example: *Next time we're in a café, what can I do to help? How can I support you to feel more confident? Shall I encourage you to do things like put the order in or pick up items we need? And what can I do if you feel stressed in the moment?*

Cheerlead

It can be tempting to focus praise on successes – the instances when our child was able to overcome avoidance. But progress in challenging anxiety will be bumpy and efforts do not always end in success. Try to take on the role of cheerleader: praise all your child's small steps and attempts irrespective of the outcome, for example saying 'well done for giving it a try', even if they do not manage the whole task as planned. The aim is to encourage your child to step into an approach-mode when they feel anxious rather than an avoid-mode. By rewarding your child whenever they step into the approach-mode, they will feel more inclined to do this next time. The risk of only rewarding success is that a child can feel inhibited about trying new things – *What if I can't manage it?* – and demoralised when an effort does not go well – *What's the point?, I'm not going to try that again.*

Be an ally

If your child does not feel able to share their difficulties with you, do not feel disheartened – not all children feel able to seek their parents' support. Do not underestimate the great help parents can offer by learning about social anxiety, giving steady support and love, and being ready if their child does want your support. Remember, most parents are not aware that their child is socially anxious.

If your child would like you to help in a more active way, that's great news.

Supporting the approach-mode

Working through this book, your child will be learning about the importance of approaching feared situations to discover how they come across and how others respond to them **in reality**, rather than based on their internal fears. This will involve doing things differently in social situations and also engaging in more social situations than they would usually. In the book we call these 'confidence tasks'. You may be able to support your child to do these.

For example:

Help planning: You might help your child to make the practical arrangements to go somewhere new or different or make the time to accompany them.

Help avoiding avoidance: This might involve gentle encouragement to take opportunities to try new things. But this can be perceived as nagging and cause conflict, so find a good moment and ask your child whether reminders/encouragement are helpful and, if so, how you should approach it.

Help doing:

• When people feel socially anxious, they become very self-conscious. Their spotlight of attention turns inwards, onto themselves. This means that they are caught up with their worries and preoccupied with their feelings of anxiety and this can make it hard for them to notice what is going on around them. When you are out and about with your child, try to encourage them to look around and notice what they can see and hear in their environment. Point out things of interest. Encourage them to become absorbed in their surroundings.

• If you are with your child in a situation, there might be particular things you could do (or not do!) to help. Ask your child in advance for guidance. When is it helpful for you to step back, when should you step in?

Help learning and building: If your child has attempted something they would typically avoid, however small, the first thing to do is praise them. Children with social anxiety can struggle to receive praise, so keep it light and low-key and give it when there isn't an audience. Ask your child to tell you what happened, keeping the emphasis on the facts and reality of what happened and away from mindreading or perceptions of what people may or may not have been thinking. Try to encourage them to think about what they have taken from the experience and make gentle suggestions if they are struggling – for example, *It suggests that you didn't stand out from the crowd, doesn't it? So maybe you come across just* *fine as you are.'* In the book you will see example confidence logs that other young people have filled in. You might want to encourage your child to use blank confidence logs to record their own learning. You could also ask what they might do next to build on their learning and how you can help. Offer suggestions if they are struggling to come up with ideas – you might find you can be playful here, perhaps making some silly suggestions to encourage your child to be creative.

Help dealing with setbacks: Setbacks are an inevitable part of the process. Young people with social anxiety will take social knocks hard. Here are some ideas of how to help your child manage and build from setbacks:

- Validate and empathise

- Remind them progress to a goal is always bumpy. Bring in your own experiences of setbacks or use examples from celebrities who resonate with your child (singers, sportspeople)

- Review what happened and see if you can spot any explanations (maybe the barista in that café is grumpy with *all* the customers?!)

- Support your child to try again

School links

School is a fundamentally social environment and so it is unsurprising that young people with social anxiety usually struggle with it. Talk to your child about if and how you might connect with their school to support them. Many children strongly refuse any engagement with their school. Use this as an opportunity for an open conversation with your child about what concerns are behind this view and how realistic they are. You may decide the best approach is to not speak to school or to engage with them. This will depend on you and your child's views about the problem, the school, and whether involving the school will help or not.

If you do agree to engage with school, then here are some topics you may want to discuss with your child first:

- How does social anxiety affect your child's time at school? Think about participating in class, speaking in front of the class, managing homework, communicating with teachers, being in the school environment generally, friendships.

- What do you or your child think might be helpful?

- Which teacher is most understanding and supportive?

- Who should speak to the teacher: you, your child or together?

Seeking professional support

Social fears are common in adolescence and for most young people these wax and wane. But, for some, the fears get in the way of everyday activities, cause significant distress and persist. If this describes your child's experience then you might consider seeking professional support. This can be important for two reasons. First, because social anxiety disorder does not tend to go away without treatment. Second, because we have treatments that work. Cognitive behavioural therapy, which is a talking treatment, is recommended. Discuss this with your child. If you do decide to seek help, speak to your GP or a teacher in school.

Caring

Knowing one's child is struggling can create anxiety, self-blame, self-doubt and worry for the future for parents. We have given lots of advice and ideas of how you might be able to help your child. But remember that you didn't 'cause' your child's anxiety and so you alone can't 'fix' it.

- **Speak to yourself kindly:** If you find you are berating yourself then try to take a breath. Ask yourself: *Is self-criticism helping?* Would you speak in this way to someone else? What would you say to another parent? Try to talk to yourself like you would a good friend. Try to give yourself encouragement and care rather than beat yourself up.

- **Seek your own support:** Talk to your partner, family, close friends.

- **Be kind to yourself:** Make time to do things that strengthen your reserves. Reading, movies, exercise, sports, cooking, shopping, listening to your favourite music. Take five minutes or an hour, whatever you can manage, and remember to build in activities that help you.

Chapter 13

Moving On

As you come to the end of this book we hope you are feeling more confident and free to be yourself. In this chapter, we will take stock of the ground covered in this book, key learning points and your plans to keep boosting your confidence. For some of you, reading this book may have helped you come to the realisation that you would like some more active help in building your confidence. We will provide some information on how to start this process.

Reviewing your goals

Go back and remind yourself of the goals you set at the start of this book (page 10):

My goals at the start were:

GOAL 1: _____

_____

_____

GOAL 2: _____

_____

_____

GOAL 3: _____

_____

_____

Take some time to think about how far you have come to reaching these goals.

Remember not to overlook all the steps you have taken, however small they might seem now. If there is still work to do, then be kind to yourself about this and think about what your next steps might be. This may involve looking into getting some further help.

Let's see what Nita noticed:

Goals at the start	My progress
GOAL 1: To answer and ask questions in class.	I don't even think about answering questions in class anymore! I do ask questions sometimes but it is something I could still do more of.
GOAL 2: To give presentations in class.	This has got much better but I have interviews coming up and I am nervous about them. So this is something I will work on.

GOAL 3: To speak up in groups and to celebrate my birthday with a group of friends this year.	I have been able to get involved in group conversations and I now enjoy them much more and also feel more connected to my friends.
GOAL 4: To allow people to take photos of me and upload selfies without filtering and editing.	I've started to enjoy wearing bright clothes and expressing myself this way now. And that includes being in photos. I'll keep working on this – on being myself more.

Now it's your turn:

Goals at the start	My progress

Now we are going to take some time to take stock and capture the helpful things you have learnt as you have worked through this book. It is a place that you can go back and look over whenever you want, especially those times when you notice your confidence wobble. It is also where you can think about further goals you might like to work towards. First, read Nita's Taking Stock summary and then have a go of filling in your own one.

Here is Nita's completed Taking Stock summary:

Where did your lack of confidence come from?
When did you first notice it? Are there any experiences that you think contributed or made it worse?

I was always a bit shy but I was OK in primary school. I found the move to secondary school hard. It felt like everyone else found their group but I didn't quite fit in. A couple of girls made comments when I spoke in class and joked about my going red. That really sticks in my mind.

What were your main negative thoughts?
I'll blush

People will think I'm a nervous wreck

They won't want to be friends with me

They'll think I'm boring

I will shake |

What have you learnt in this book?

Refresh yourself by looking at the different chapters. What did you find helpful? What has stuck with you?

I don't look as red as I feel

Even if I do look red, other people don't notice or judge

People like me as I am

I learnt to get out of my head and focus on the situation

I learnt to test my fears out using confidence experiments

I learnt to speak kindly to myself

I don't shake as much as I feel I do

Shaking isn't on other people's radar

How will you deal with setbacks?

What kind of things might set you back or knock your confidence? What will you do to get back on track? Think about the skills you have learnt in this book that might help.

A setback for me would be applying for a part-time job but not being offered it.

I would deal with it by:

Looking back at the 'be kind to myself' chapter to make sure I don't dwell on it.

Talk to my mum.

Plan some confidence experiments.

350 Overcoming Social Anxiety and Building Self-confidence

How will you build on your progress?

What are your next steps for building your confidence? Are you still avoiding anything or hiding away? Are there opportunities you could make the most of?

I am planning on applying for a part-time job. I will ask my mum to look over my CV and to do a practice interview with me. I plan to go to a concert with my friends this summer and I am going to wear my favourite colourful outfit and we will take lots of pictures of ourselves. I couldn't have imagined even considering this before!

Now you can take some time to take stock.

Taking stock

> **Where did your lack of confidence come from?**
>
> When did you first notice it? Are there any experiences that you think contributed or made it worse?

> **What were your main negative thoughts?**

> **What kept them going?**
>
> Think about self-focus, behaviour traps and the feelings and images you relied on to judge how you came across.

What have you learnt in this book?

Refresh yourself by looking at the different chapters. What did you find helpful? What has stuck with you?

How will you deal with setbacks?

What kind of things might set you back or knock your confidence? What will you do to get back on track? Think about the skills you have learnt in this book that might help.

> **How will you build on your progress?**
>
> What are your next steps for building your confidence? Are you still avoiding anything or hiding away? Are there opportunities you could make the most of?

Need a bit more support?

Reading this book may have helped you to realise that you would like more active help to feel better in social situations. If that is the case, then the best way to do it is by talking to someone. We have guidance on how to talk to other people in order to get some help in Chapter 12, Helping Others Help Me. The good news is that there are excellent treatments available that will help you overcome social anxiety. The treatments with the best evidence are a type of talking therapy called cognitive behavioural therapy (or CBT). Your family or teacher at school will be able to direct you to the right help.

Well done on working your way through this book! Facing up to our struggles head on is never easy. Remember, we all feel anxious and doubt ourselves at times. It is part of being human. We hope you can give yourself a huge amount of credit for getting this far. Wherever you are on your journey towards building self-confidence and however many steps you still have to go, we wish you the best and hope you can be kind to yourself. Our greatest hope is that going forward you can use what you have learnt here to start being yourself more around others. Take things step by step. Getting out of your head and sharing more of your wonderful self with others is ultimately the route to feeling more socially confident and building better connections.

Resources

In this section are resources and links that we have referred to in the book and which you might find helpful when you are trying out activities to build your social confidence.

Mapping my social anxiety

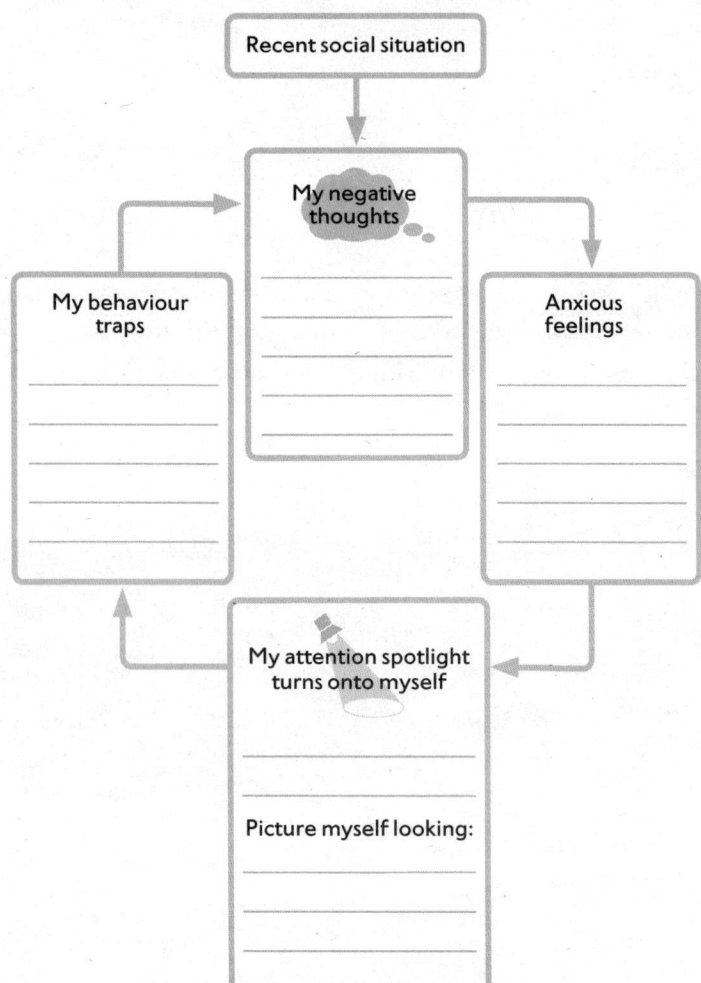

Mapping my social anxiety

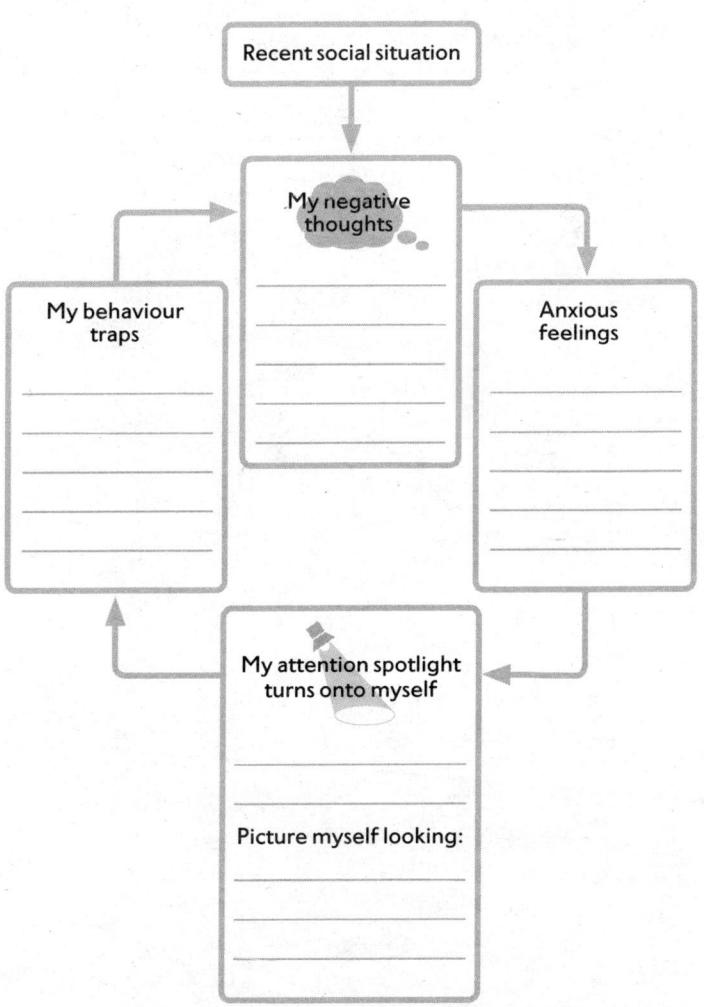

Confidence Experiment Log

Step 1. Belief	Step 2. Situation	Step 3. Predict	Step 4. Do it!	Step 5. Reflect	Step 6. Look ahead	
What fearful belief will you focus on?	*What situation will you test out your fear in?*	*What is the worst that you think might happen?* *How would you know? 0–100%*	*How will you test it out?* *Remember to get externally focused and drop behaviour traps.*	*What happened?* *Re-rate your prediction (0–100%).* *What does this tell you about yourself more generally?*	*What are you going to try next to build on your learning?*	

Taking stock

Where did your lack of confidence come from?

When did you first notice it? Are there any experiences that you think contributed or made it worse?

What were your main negative thoughts?

What kept them going?

Think about self-focus, behaviour traps and the feelings and images you relied on to judge how you came across.

What have you learnt in this book?

Refresh yourself by looking at the different chapters. What did you find helpful? What has stuck with you?

How will you deal with setbacks?

What kind of things might set you back or knock your confidence? What will you do to get back on track? Think about the skills you have learnt in this book that might help.

How will you build on your progress?

What are your next steps for building your confidence? Are you still avoiding anything or hiding away? Are there opportunities you could make the most of?

Virtual Audiences

Use this link to access the 'virtual audiences': https://www.youtube.com/playlist?list=PLjGQ1qp_lGNUOjLW60dkID x7qs0jSuA9c

A virtual audience is a pre-recorded video of people listening to a talk or presentation. We have several different-sized virtual audiences online. Some are more challenging than others because they look less engaged with the speaker. You may want to start with the standard audience of three and build up to a larger, more challenging audience. We have found that doing this can start to build confidence in public speaking. Importantly, drop those behaviour traps and focus on the task at hand, rather than yourself!

Online Resources

Link: https://overcoming.co.uk/715/resources-to-download

e-versions of therapy materials available:

- Mapping my own anxiety

- Confidence experiment log

- Taking stock summary

- A family's guide to social anxiety

- Information about virtual audiences with link

Index

Note: page numbers in **bold** refer to diagrams.